Robotic Surgery

Go Watanabe
Editor

Robotic Surgery

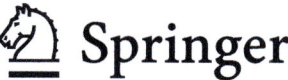

Editor
Go Watanabe
Department of General and Cardiothoracic Surgery
Kanazawa University
Ishikawa, Japan

ISBN 978-4-431-54852-2   ISBN 978-4-431-54853-9 (eBook)
DOI 10.1007/978-4-431-54853-9
Springer Tokyo Heidelberg New York Dordrecht London

Library of Congress Control Number: 2014934698

© Springer Japan 2014

This work is subject to copyright. All rights are reserved by the Publisher, whether the whole or part of the material is concerned, specifically the rights of translation, reprinting, reuse of illustrations, recitation, broadcasting, reproduction on microfilms or in any other physical way, and transmission or information storage and retrieval, electronic adaptation, computer software, or by similar or dissimilar methodology now known or hereafter developed. Exempted from this legal reservation are brief excerpts in connection with reviews or scholarly analysis or material supplied specifically for the purpose of being entered and executed on a computer system, for exclusive use by the purchaser of the work. Duplication of this publication or parts thereof is permitted only under the provisions of the Copyright Law of the Publisher's location, in its current version, and permission for use must always be obtained from Springer. Permissions for use may be obtained through RightsLink at the Copyright Clearance Center. Violations are liable to prosecution under the respective Copyright Law.

The use of general descriptive names, registered names, trademarks, service marks, etc. in this publication does not imply, even in the absence of a specific statement, that such names are exempt from the relevant protective laws and regulations and therefore free for general use.

While the advice and information in this book are believed to be true and accurate at the date of publication, neither the authors nor the editors nor the publisher can accept any legal responsibility for any errors or omissions that may be made. The publisher makes no warranty, express or implied, with respect to the material contained herein.

Printed on acid-free paper

Springer is part of Springer Science+Business Media (www.springer.com)

Preface

It is a great honor to serve as editor for this book of robotic surgery.

The da Vinci Surgical System was first launched in 1999. In the beginning, the device was marketed with major features that included fine tissue manipulation capability, such as in coronary artery bypass grafting. Gradually the efficacy of its multidimensional forceps and three-dimensional endoscope was increasingly applied to diverse diseases outside the cardiac field. Notably, robot-assisted surgery is becoming the gold standard for urological surgeries including prostatectomy. Furthermore, gynecology has been recognized as the next main focus, and "national diseases" including digestive diseases in Asian countries have also become the target of application. Regarding cardiac surgeries, the da Vinci system is currently used in coronary artery bypass grafting by a limited number of surgeons because of the complicated techniques involved, but applications to structural heart diseases such as valvular diseases and atrial septal defect are expanding. In these ways, robotics has made revolutionary changes to the future of surgery in all surgical disciplines. Since Billroth conducted the first successful gastrectomy, there have been few landmarks of progress in the history of surgery. However, accompanying the introduction of the da Vinci system, we are witnessing a gradual shift of all surgical treatments to endoscopic and robot-assisted procedures. This book summarizes the current developments together with updates.

I have invited leading experts in their respective fields to write the chapters of this book and to share with us the most up-to-date knowledge. I would like to express my gratitude to all the authors for their valuable contributions.

Ishikawa, Japan Go Watanabe
November 2013

Contents

1. **Overview of Robotic Surgery** 1
   Kenoki Ohuchida and Makoto Hashizume

2. **The da Vinci Surgical® Systems** 9
   M.E. Hagen and M.J. Curet

3. **Development of Robotic Systems** 21
   M.E. Hagen and M.J. Curet

4. **Robotic Surgery in Urology** 31
   Masaaki Tachibana and Kunihiko Yoshioka

5. **Robotic Gastrectomy for Gastric Cancer** 49
   Kazutaka Obama and Woo Jin Hyung

6. **Esophageal Cancer Surgery: Robotic Esophagectomy in the Prone Position** 63
   Koichi Suda and Ichiro Uyama

7. **Lateral Pelvic Node Dissection for Advanced Rectal Cancer: Current Debates and Use of the Robotic Approach** 75
   Gyu-Seog Choi

8. **Cardiac Surgery: Overview** 87
   Go Watanabe

9. **Robotically Assisted Totally Endoscopic Coronary Artery Bypass Grafting** 97
   Johannes Bonatti, Stephanie Mick, Nikolaos Bonaros,
   Eric Lehr, Ravi Nair, and Tomislav Mihaljevic

10. **Robotic Surgery for Mitral Valve Disease** 111
    Tsuyoshi Kaneko, Bryan Bush, Wiley Nifong,
    and W. Randolph Chitwood Jr.

11 **Robotic Surgery in General Thoracic Surgery** 121
Hyun-Sung Lee and Hee-Jin Jang

12 **Robot-Assisted Thyroidectomy** 145
Norihiko Ishikawa

Overview of Robotic Surgery

Kenoki Ohuchida and Makoto Hashizume

1.1 The Development of Robotic Surgical System

More than 25 years ago, robotic surgical system was introduced in the surgical field. In 1985, Kwoh et al. [17] modified industrial robot and performed biopsies in the neurosurgical field using the modified robot. In this surgical procedure, the modified robot provided the greater precision than the conventional procedure. In 1993, AESOP™ (Automated Endoscopic System for Optimal Positioning), which had pedals or voice-controlled robotic arm with an endoscope, was developed by Computer Motion Inc. (Goleta, CA, USA) and the Food and Drug Administration (FDA) approved the fist model of the AESOP™ in 1994. This system made it possible for the surgeon to control his visual field. In 1992, as the active robot, the ROBODOC™ (ISS, Integrated Surgical Systems, Sacramento, CA, USA) was developed for total hip replacement in the orthopedic field [5]. This system provided the precision of the milling of the femoral cavity with the program based on the preoperative imaging and the perioperative information. In 2008, FDA approved a revised ROBODOC™ system (Curexo Technology Corp., Fremont, CA, USA), which is now commercially available in the USA.

As the master–slave system, ZEUS™ robotic surgical system was introduced by Computer Motion Inc. (Goleta, CA, USA) in 1998 and improved surgeon dexterity in the minimally invasive surgery. ZEUS™ consisted of two physically separated subsystems, which were a surgeon control center and three robotic arms attached to the operating table. The computer system in ZEUS connects the surgeon control center and robotic arms and can filter tremors and provide 3D vision [12]. In 2001, Marescaux et al. [18] used ZEUS™ system to perform the first transatlantic robot-assisted laparoscopic cholecystectomy between New York and Strasburg using a

---

K. Ohuchida • M. Hashizume (✉)
Department of Advanced Medical Initiatives, Graduate School of Medical Sciences, Kyushu University, Fukuoka, Japan
e-mail: mhashi@dem.med.kyushu-u.ac.jp

high-speed connection. The ZEUS™ system was also used in cardiovascular surgery, gynecologic surgery, digestive surgery, and urologic surgery for several years [8]. However, the development of the ZEUS™ system was stopped because the Intuitive Surgical Inc. (Mountain View, CA, USA) acquired Computer Motion Inc.

1.2 The da Vinci™ Surgical System

The da Vinci™ Surgical System with 3D vision was developed by Intuitive Surgical (Mountain View, CA). In 1997, Himens and Cadiere performed the first robot-assisted cholecystectomy using the prototype of the da Vinci™ Surgical System [9]. In 2000, FDA approved the da Vinci™ Surgical System for general laparoscopic surgery. In 2002, FDA approved the modified version of this system with a fourth robotic arm. Intuitive Surgical introduced the da Vinci S system and the da Vinci Si system in 2006 and 2009, respectively. Especially, the da Vinci Si system provides 3D full high-definition vision system and the second console for training.

Today, the da Vinci™ Surgical System is the only commercially available master–slave robotic system. So far, more than 2,300 da Vinci systems have been installed worldwide. Many kinds of surgical operations, such as general surgery [10, 11], gynecologic surgery, urologic surgery, pediatric surgery, cardiothoracic surgery, and other operations [24], were performed using the da Vinci™ Surgical System.

The da Vinci™ Surgical System was composed of three main parts including the surgeon console, the surgical cart with one camera arm and three arms directly performing the procedures, and the 3D imaging system. The surgeon console has the computer system to control the whole system. One of the features of the da Vinci™ Surgical System is visualization through a high-quality 3D endoscope. Another one of the features is the surgical instrument with the EndoWrist™, which mimics human hand motion by artificial articulation. The da Vinci™ Surgical System provides surgeons with an intuitive translation of the instrument handle to the tip movement, thus avoiding the mirror-image effect. In addition, this system is equipped with tremor filtering, scaling function, and coaxial alignment of the eyes, hand, and tooltip image. Furthermore, an internal articulated endoscopic wrist in this system provides an additional three degrees of freedom. To date, in the surgical treatment of cancers or tumors, surgeons need more intricate dissection with oncological approaches. Using the da Vinci™ Surgical System, we had successfully performed robotic surgery for gastric cancer, esophageal tumors, retromediastinal tumor, thymoma, and colon cancer [7, 11, 24].

In order for robotic surgery to spread more widely, however, there are several basic problems that remain to be resolved. One of them is the price of surgical robots. Depending on the countries and insurance systems, medical insurance coverage for robotic surgery is limited. The downsizing of robotic system and the development of navigation systems to support robotic surgery are also needed. Furthermore, the lack of training systems for surgeons is an important problem.

In this point, several institutes have reported an excellent testimony to the significance of training [1, 22]. In July 2003, we also established the Center for Integration of Advanced Medicine, Life Science and Innovative Technology (CAMIT) at Kyushu University and started a training course, which is called "Hands-on Training for Robotic Surgery at Kyushu University." There were two training courses for robotic surgery. One was a two-day course with an animate laboratory and the other was a one-day inanimate laboratory course. Both courses were open, not only to medical doctors but also to a wider range of engineering researchers in both industry and academia.

1.3 Perspective of Robotic Surgery

1.3.1 Robotic Single-Port Surgery

Laparoscopic surgery has several advantages over conventional open surgery. Laparoscopic surgery significantly contributes decreased postoperative pain, shortened hospital stay, and effective magnification of the surgical view. Three to six ports are usually used depending on the operations in laparoscopic surgery. However, the use of multiple ports leads to the increase in the potential chance of morbidity from port-site hernia, bleeding, and internal organ damage as well as to the decrease in the cosmetic outcome. Single-port or single-incision laparoscopic surgery is one of the emerging concepts. In the single-port surgery, all of the laparoscopic working ports are entered through the abdominal or chest wall via the same incision. This surgery contributes to excellent cosmesis, and the surgical scar is often undetectable. Especially, there seems to be no scar when it has been concealed within the umbilicus. Recently, from an oncological prognostic standpoint, the potential advantages of single-port surgery for the surgical treatment of cancers include comparable results to the conventional laparoscopic procedure and an open procedure.

In single-port surgery, the multiple instruments and laparoscopes compete for the same space at the fulcrum of the entry port, especially in the case of advanced surgery. Furthermore, in the external area, the collision of surgeon's hands greatly causes the limitation of the internal manipulation of the instrument tips. One of the potential solutions to this problem is the use of a surgical robotic system. A robotic system can switch the right- and left-handed instruments on the control panel. And it makes the surgeon manipulate the crossed instruments on the console as they would if they were not crossed. Furthermore, compared with the laparoscopic surgery with multiple ports, a robotic system offers advantages, such as range of motion, three-dimensional visualization, and scaling of movement that is superior to that of conventional laparoscopic surgery.

The robotic system has already been introduced into single-port laparoscopic surgery. The first clinical cases with robotic single-port surgery were reported in urology patients who received a radical prostatectomy, a radical nephrectomy, and a dismembered pyeloplasty [14]. Additionally, a partial cecectomy, a hysterectomy [20], and a right colectomy [19] have been performed with robotic single-port surgery. The combination of single-port laparoscopic surgery and the existing robotic system will provide surgical benefits without the increase in the complications or conversion to laparotomy. However, the current robotic system is not specifically designed for single-port surgery. Recently, Intuitive Surgical Inc. has developed new version of instruments and trocars, which are semirigid, for robotic single-port surgery. These instruments are inserted thorough curved trocars to avoid the collisions between robotic arms. Although further optimization of the robotic system [15, 16] for single-port surgery was reported, further prospective studies will be needed to expand the robotic single-port surgery throughout the world.

1.3.2 Robotic Natural Orifice Transluminal Endoscopic Surgery

Natural orifice transluminal endoscopic surgery (NOTES) is a less invasive surgery without any scars. In this procedure, an endoscope is inserted through a natural orifice, such as the mouth, vagina, anus, or the urethral opening. Then, this endoscope penetrates a luminal wall such as the gastric, colonic, rectal, vaginal, or vesicle wall to move into the abdominal cavity for the diagnosis or the surgical treatment of target internal organs. Kalloo et al. reported the use of NOTES in the first animal study in 2004 [13] and Rao et al. performed the first human case of NOTES in India. NOTES seems to be less invasive than conventional laparoscopic surgery and possibly contributes to faster postoperative recovery and return to normal activities than conventional laparoscopic surgery. Because NOTES leaves no postoperative scar on the abdomen, the incidence of complications related to abdominal wall incisions including infections, bleeding, and postoperative incisional hernias can be decreased. However, NOTES is still in the experimental phase. In NOTES, to perform the surgical procedures, surgeons must manipulate endoscopic forceps through the conventional flexible endoscopic channel alone. It is not easy to provide the degree of maneuverability required for the excision of the abdominal organs such as the appendix and the gallbladder.

The application of robotic technology is one of the solutions to this problem. A robotic system can be applied to enable the versatile manipulation of endoscopic forceps in a narrow visual field and a small cavity. It has been reported that the robotic system was used for NOTES in clinics [6]. When forceps that can be manipulated through a tight, small-diameter, flexible endoscopic channel are developed, robotic NOTES will be a more promising approach. In Kyushu University, we have several projects to develop a robotic system for use with NOTES. One of them has also been in progress with the development of small multijoint arms. We are also developing NOTES-dedicated endoscopic system equipped with an ultrasound diagnosis/treatment device. This robotic NOTES system is designed to have a large forceps channel to allow for a better manipulation, a higher illumination light intensity, a wider viewing angle, and a higher-resolution display than

1 Overview of Robotic Surgery

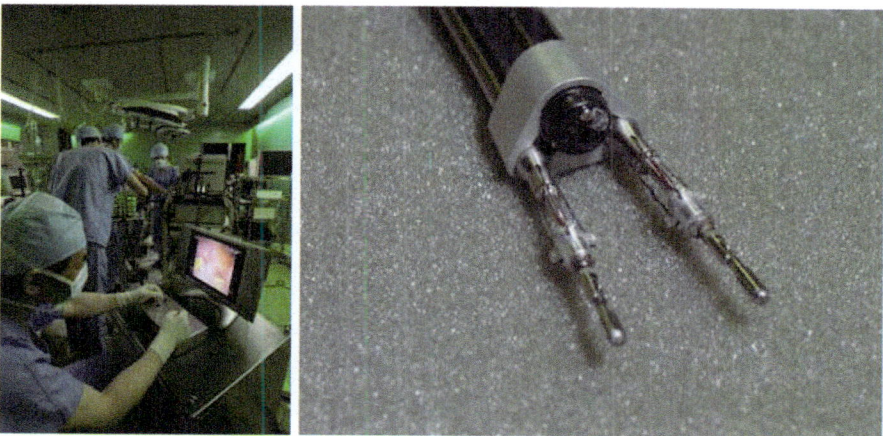

Fig. 1.1 Endoscopic robot system for NOTES

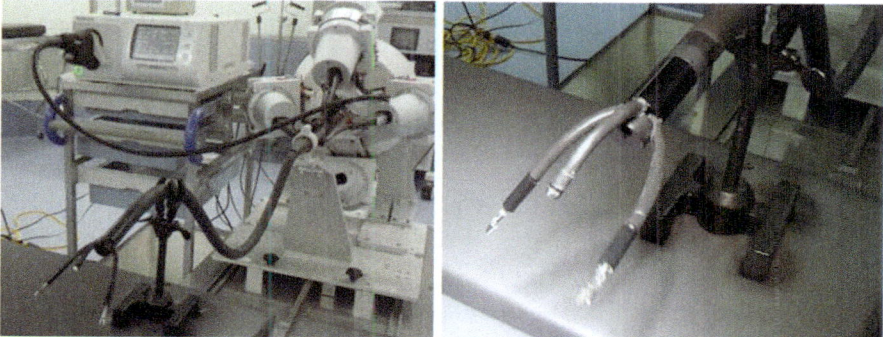

Fig. 1.2 Flexible endoscope with two robotic arms

the conventional flexible endoscopic systems. A master–slave surgical robot for NOTES (Figs. 1.1 and 1.2) also has been developed at Kyushu University [3, 23]. Such application of robotic technology is therefore expected to significantly contribute to the widespread use of NOTES.

1.4 Conclusion

Although the advantages and disadvantages of a robotic system have been discussed, the further development of equipment and technologies is essential to allow the safe, widespread adoption of a robotic system in minimally invasive surgery, especially in more advanced surgery for malignant tumors, single-port surgery, and NOTES. Robotic system also contributes to telesurgery or remote surgery [2]. Therefore, in the future, robotic system will make it possible to perform surgical procedure in the battlefield or the outer space without sending surgeons. The combination between robotic surgery and navigation surgery is also promising because of the use of 3D data and the easy recognition of the tip of robotic arm and endoscope. In the present robotic surgery, it is difficult to collaborate with surgical assistants because of the large scale of robotic arms. It is also a large problem to take a long time to set up for robotic system. The future downsizing of robotic system may resolve such problems. Although there are other problems facing the medical use of a robotic system, the da Vinci™ Surgical System has already been used all over the world. Advances in the medical field of robotics will hopefully overcome these problems and provide the ultimate minimally invasive surgery.

References

1. Amodeo A, Linares Quevedo A, Joseph JV, Belgrano E, Patel HR (2009) Robotic laparoscopic surgery: cost and training [Review]. Minerva Urol Nefrol (Ital J Urol Nephrol) 61(2):121–128
2. Arata J, Takahashi H, Pitakwatchara P, Warisawa S, Tanoue K, Konishi K, Ieiri S, Shimizu S, Nakashima N, Okamura K, Fujino Y, Ueda Y, Chotiwan P, Mitsuishi M, Hashizume M (2007) A remote surgery experiment between Japan and Thailand over internet using a low latency CODEC system. In: IEEE international conference on robotics and automation, Roma, Italy, pp 10–14
3. Arata J, Kenmotsu H, Takagi M, Hori T, Miyagi T, Fujimoto H, Kajita Y, Hayashi Y, Chinzei K, Hashizume M (2013) Surgical bedside master console for neurosurgical robotic system. Int J Comput Assist Radiol Surg 8(1):75–86
4. Ballantyne GH (2002) Robotic surgery, telerobotic surgery, telepresence, and telementoring. Review of early clinical results [Review]. Surg Endosc 16(10):1389–1402
5. Cowley G (1992) Introducing "Robodoc". A robot finds his calling: in the operating room. Newsweek 120(21):86
6. Haber GP, Crouzet S, Kamoi K, Berger A, Aron M, Goel R et al (2008) Robotic NOTES (natural orifice translumenal endoscopic surgery) in reconstructive urology: initial laboratory experience [Evaluation studies]. Urology 71(6):996–1000
7. Hashizume M, Sugimachi K (2003) Robot-assisted gastric surgery. Surg Clin North Am 83(6):1429–1444
8. Hashizume M, Konishi K, Tsutsumi N, Yamaguchi S, Shimabukuro R (2002) A new era of robotic surgery assisted by a computer-enhanced surgical system [Review]. Surgery 131(1 Suppl):S330–S333
9. Himpens J, Leman G, Cadiere GB (1998) Telesurgical laparoscopic cholecystectomy [Case reports letter]. Surg Endosc 12(8):1091
10. Isogaki J, Haruta S, Man IM, Suda K, Kawamura Y, Yoshimura F et al (2011) Robot-assisted surgery for gastric cancer: experience at our institute. Pathobiol J Immunopathol Mol Cell Biol 78(6):328–333
11. Kakeji Y, Konishi K, Ieiri S, Yasunaga T, Nakamoto M, Tanoue K et al (2006) Robotic laparoscopic distal gastrectomy: a comparison of the da Vinci and Zeus systems. [Comparative study evaluation studies research support, Non-U.S. gov't]. Int J Med Robot Comput Assist Surg (MRCAS) 2(4):299–304

12. Kalan I, Turgut D, Aksoy S, Dede DS, Dizdar O, Ozisik Y et al (2010) Clinical and pathological characteristics of breast cancer patients with history of cesarean delivery [Letter]. Breast 19(1):67–68
13. Kalloo AN, Singh VK, Jagannath SB, Niiyama H, Hill SL, Vaughn CA et al (2004) Flexible transgastric peritoneoscopy: a novel approach to diagnostic and therapeutic interventions in the peritoneal cavity. [Research support, Non-U.S. gov't]. Gastrointest Endosc 60(1):114–117
14. Kaouk JH, Goel RK, Haber GP, Crouzet S, Stein RJ (2009) Robotic single-port transumbilical surgery in humans: initial report [Evaluation studies]. BJU Int 103(3):366–369
15. Kobayashi Y, Sekiguchi Y, Tomono Y, Watanabe H, Toyoda K, Konishi K et al. (2010) Design of a surgical robot with dynamic vision field control for single port endoscopic surgery [Research support, Non-U.S. Gov't]. In: Conference proceedings: annual international conference of the IEEE engineering in medicine and biology society, Buenos Aires, Argentina, pp 979–983
16. Kobayashi Y, Tomono Y, Sekiguchi Y, Watanabe H, Toyoda K, Konishi K et al (2010) A surgical robot with vision field control for single port endoscopic surgery [Research support, Non-U.S. gov't]. Int J Med Robot Comput Assist Surg (MRCAS) 6(4):454–464
17. Kwoh YS, Hou J, Jonckheere EA, Hayati S (1988) A robot with improved absolute positioning accuracy for CT guided stereotactic brain surgery. IEEE Trans Biomed Eng 35(2):153–160
18. Marescaux J, Leroy J, Gagner M, Rubino F, Mutter D, Vix M et al (2001) Transatlantic robot-assisted telesurgery. Nature 413(6854):379–380
19. Ostrowitz MB, Eschete D, Zemon H, DeNoto G (2009) Robotic-assisted single-incision right colectomy: early experience. Int J Med Robot Comput Assist Surg (MRCAS) 5(4):465–470
20. Ragupathi M, Ramos-Valadez DI, Pedraza R, Haas EM (2010) Robotic-assisted single-incision laparoscopic partial cececctomy [Case reports]. Int J Med Robot Comput Assist Surg (MRCAS) 6(3):362–367
21. Reynolds W Jr (2001) The first laparoscopic cholecystectomy [Biography historical article portraits]. JSLS 5(1):89–94
22. Suh I, Mukherjee M, Oleynikov D, Su KC (2011) Training program for fundamental surgical skill in robotic laparoscopic surgery. Int J Med Robot Comput Assist Surg (MRCAS) 7(3):327–333
23. Suzuki N, Hattori A, Ieiri S, Konishi K, Maeda T, Fujino Y, Ueda Y, Navicharern P, Tanoue K, Hashizume M (2009) Tele-control of an endoscopic surgical robot system between Japan and Thailand for tele-NOTES. Stud Health Technol Inform 142:374–379
24. Yoshino I, Hashizume M, Shimada M, Tomikawa M, Sugimachi K (2002) Video-assisted thoracoscopic extirpation of a posterior mediastinal mass using the da Vinci computer enhanced surgical system [Case reports]. Ann Thorac Surg 74(4):1235–1237

The da Vinci Surgical® Systems

M.E. Hagen and M.J. Curet

2.1 Historical Overview

The da Vinci® Surgical System (Intuitive Surgical Inc., Sunnyvale, CA, USA) is at present the most commonly used robotic system for performing minimally invasive laparoscopic surgery in humans.

Currently, the system is cleared by the Food and Drug Administration (FDA) for the use in urological surgical procedures, general laparoscopic surgical procedures, gynecologic laparoscopic surgical procedures, transoral otolaryngology surgical procedures restricted to benign and malignant tumors classified as T1 and T2, general thoracoscopic surgical procedures, and thoracoscopically assisted cardiotomy procedures. The system has also received clearance to be employed with adjunctive mediastinotomy to perform coronary anastomosis during cardiac revascularization. It is indicated for adult and pediatric use—with the exception of transoral otolaryngology surgical procedures in pediatric patients (as of December 2012). Additionally, the da Vinci Surgical System is cleared for a variety of indications in large part of Europe, Asia, and other parts of the world.

During the late 1980s, a number of scientific groups worldwide developed robotic surgery research projects in an effort to overcome some of the most common challenges of conventional surgical techniques. Early funding to several of these teams was provided by the Defense Advanced Research Projects Agency (DARPA)—amongst these was the former Stanford Research Institute, now known as SRI International, which provided the basis for the development of the da Vinci® Surgical System. The original interest of the US army was to develop a telesurgical system that would enable remote battlefield surgical care. However, further

---

M.E. Hagen • M.J. Curet (✉)
Intuitive Surgical, Inc., 1266 Kifer Road, Building 101, Sunnyvale, CA 94086-5304, USA
e-mail: Myriam.Curet@intusurg.com

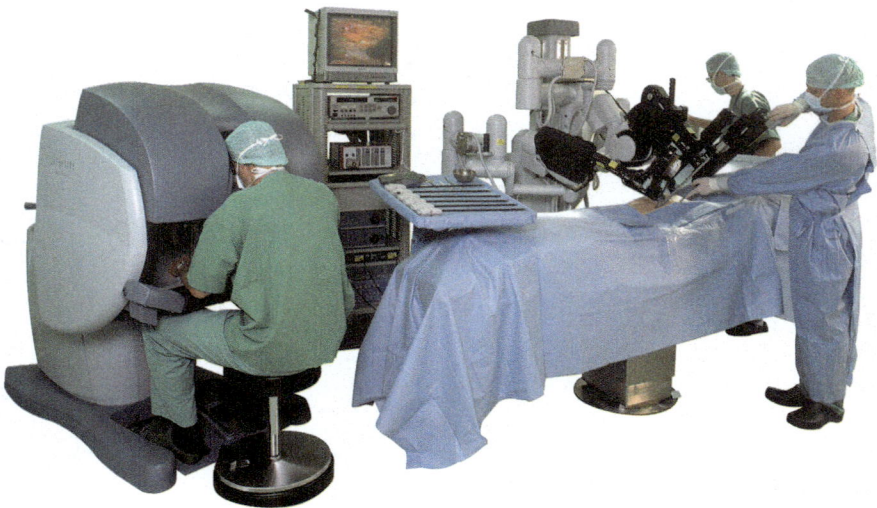

Fig. 2.1 The da Vinci® Standard Surgical System

investigations of the group revealed that a civilian use would by far outshine the use of an exclusive military application by accelerating the applications of minimally invasive surgery to a far wider range of more complex procedures.

Driven by this purpose, Intuitive Surgical was founded in 1995. The main purpose of the company has been to develop a reliable, intuitive, surgical device that would deliver the benefits of minimally invasive surgery to the patient while preserving the benefits of open surgery for the operator. Specifically, the technology was designed to address the limitations of conventional laparoscopy by improving the ergonomics, dexterity, and visualization.

The early efforts of Intuitive Surgical resulted in the ancestor of the current da Vinci® Surgical System. This first system was named "Lenny" and was used exclusively for animal testing. These experiments confirmed the value of wristed instruments as an integral element of minimally invasive surgery. The next generation was named "Mona" and was used in the first human trials in 1997 in Belgium for a variety of abdominal procedures. These early experiences lead to the design of the first "da Vinci" Standard Surgical System (Fig. 2.1), which was launched in Europe in January 1999 and received FDA clearance in the USA for general laparoscopic surgery in 2000.

As of the end of 2012, more than 2,500 da Vinci Surgical® Systems have been installed in over 2,000 hospitals worldwide. Intuitive Surgical remains the market leader for robotic minimally invasive surgery by holding the exclusive field-of-use license for more than 1,000 US and foreign patents that cover the important aspects of its technology including the surgical console, the vision system, and the wristed instruments.

2.2 The da Vinci® Models

There have been three commercial models of the da Vinci Surgical System: the da Vinci® Standard System, the da Vinci® S System (Fig. 2.2), and the most current version, the da Vinci Si® Surgical System (Fig. 2.3). All three share the main components that characterize this family of tele-manipulators: a surgical console, a surgical cart, and a vision cart.

However, significant improvements have been integrated over the years. The da Vinci® Standard System has been discontinued from sale and is no longer supported by Intuitive Surgical, although a few models are still in use, mainly in laboratories and research centers. The second version, the da Vinci® S Surgical System, was designed to facilitate surgical setup through a slimmer arm design and the addition of a fourth robotic arm. The types and sizes of available wristed instruments were expanded, including the addition of longer instruments that allow for greater reach within the abdominal cavity. This version was also equipped with high-definition (HD) video and an improved user interface. The latest product iteration—the da Vinci® Si Surgical System—was released to the international market in 2009 and features two control consoles that can be used in tandem, the addition of an integrated laser technology to allow for fluorescent imaging and single-site technology. The dual-console setup allows for two surgeons to collaborate during surgery, for at-console case observation and for telementoring. A further enhancement with this version is the addition of a surgical simulator, which can be attached to the back of the surgical console for training and demonstration purposes.

A detailed description of the latest da Vinci Si Surgical System follows:

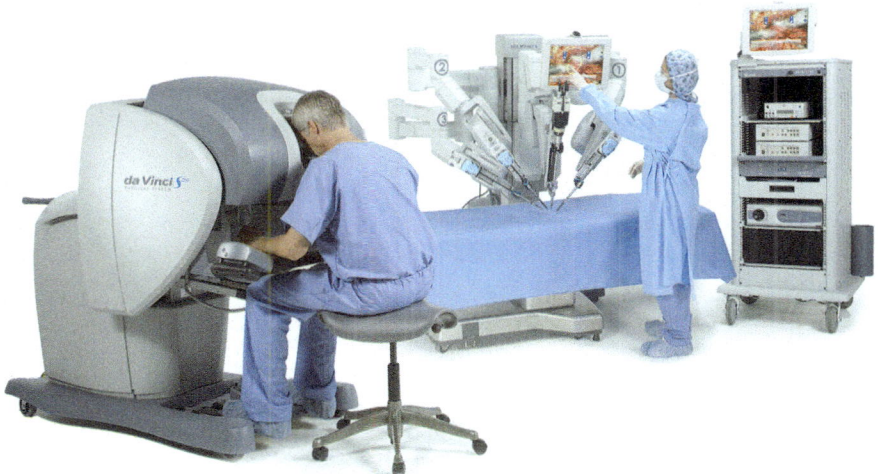

Fig. 2.2 The da Vinci® S Surgical System

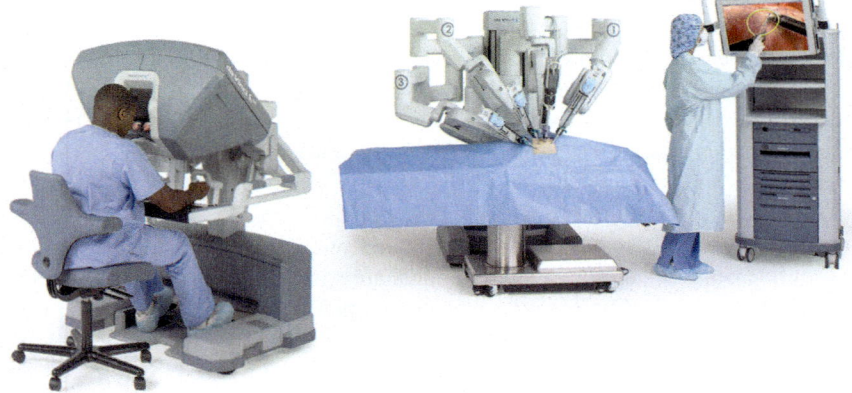

Fig. 2.3 The da Vinci® Si Surgical System

Fig. 2.4 The surgical console

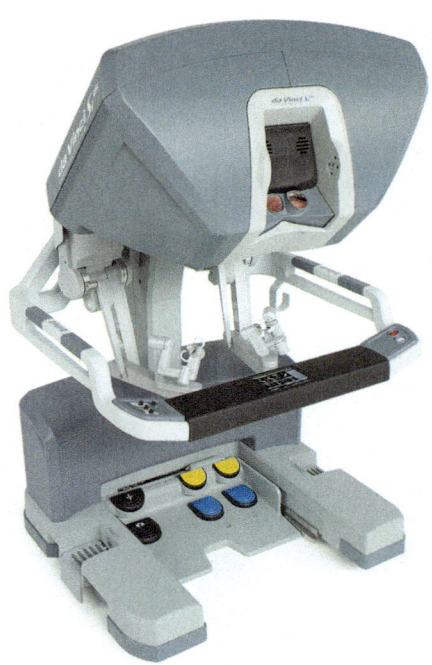

2.2.1 The da Vinci® Components: The Surgical Console

The surgeon console (Fig. 2.4) is the central control component of the da Vinci Si System and includes the master controllers, the stereo viewer, the central touch pad, the left and right pods, and the footswitch panel. The operating surgeon sits at the

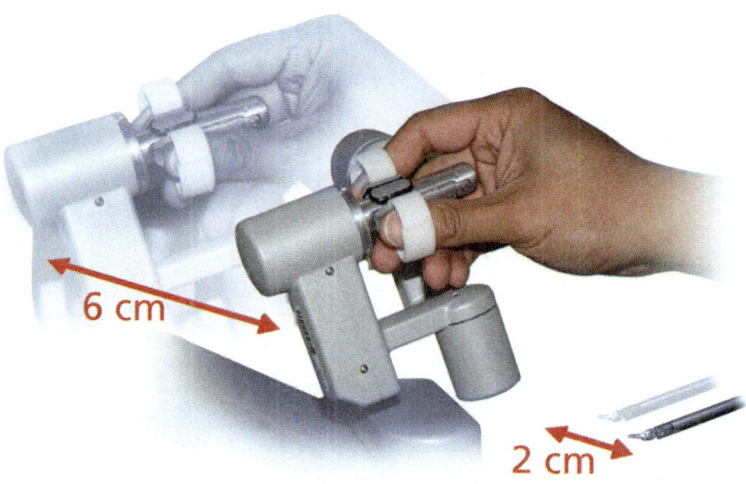

Fig. 2.5 The da Vinci® master controllers

console, which is outside of the sterile field, and controls the movements of the robotic arms, the 3D endoscope, and the EndoWrist® instruments. The surgical image is streamed real time into the stereo viewer, where instruments appear to align with the master controllers and thus with the surgeon's hands. This important concept is called the anthropomorphic principle and means that the motion capabilities of the da Vinci arms and instruments are designed to mimic those of its human operator. Whenever possible, the limits of the system coincide with the human hand, which results in a natural alignment of the eye, hand, and surgical instrument. This design leverages surgical dexterity that is comparable to open surgery but in a minimally invasive setup.

The *master controllers* (Fig. 2.5) are the manual control units of the surgeon and work very similarly to computer joy-sticks. They are designed so that the left and right hand can each control a robotic arm and the instrument mounted on it. The master controllers contain finger grips and wrist and elbow/shoulder joints so that the movements of the designated instrument within the surgical field mimic the movements of the surgeon's hand, wrist, thumb, and index or middle finger, supporting the anthropomorphic principle. Clutch buttons that disengage the master controllers from the robotic instruments can be operated with an additional finger. These clutch buttons enable repositioning of the master controllers without robotic arm or instrument movement.

The *stereo viewer* is the central visual element of the robotic system and allows the user to view the surgical site in 3D, as well as to access additional information via icons and text messages. This system allows the surgeon to choose between a full-screen mode and a multi-image mode. The multi-image or TilePro™ mode displays the image of the surgical field along with up to two additional images such as a CT scan according to the surgeon's choice (Fig. 2.6). The images displayed in

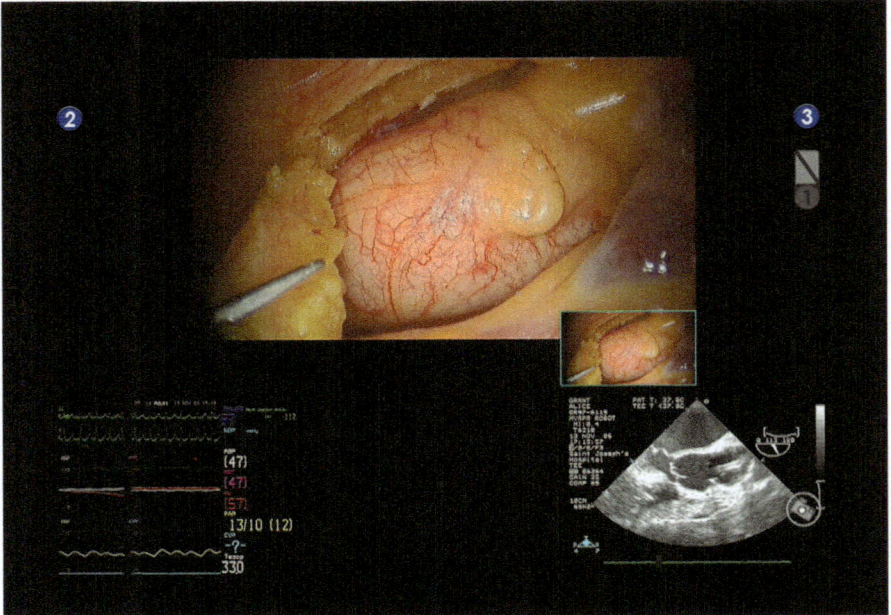

Fig. 2.6 TilePro™ mode

the stereo viewer are duplicated on a monitor mounted on the vision cart for the bedside personnel. The stereo viewer is located immediately below the headrest, which also contains a microphone and a pair of speakers. The monitor mounted on the vision cart also contains a microphone and speakers, allowing for smooth two-way verbal communication between the console surgeon and the additional personnel at the bedside.

The central *touchpad* is an important system control unit of the surgical console. The home screen of the touchpad displays the system status, and buttons on the touchpad control the scope angle, the zoom level, and the motion scaling. Instrument arm selection and dual-console configuration—assigning robotic arm control between the two consoles—are also performed using the touchpad.

The *left and right side pods* are control panels located on either side of the master controllers. The *left side pod* controls ergonomic adjustments, which is particularly important to avoid physical strain during long surgical procedures. The *right side pod* is equipped with power and emergency stop buttons.

The *footswitch panel* (Fig. 2.7) allows the surgeon to swap control of the robotic arms between the master controllers, to swap control from the endoscopic instruments to the camera, to control the master clutch, and to activate primary and secondary energy sources. The footswitch panel is found directly beneath the surgeon and is controlled by the surgeon's feet.

Two surgical consoles can be used simultaneously with a single surgical cart—in the so-called *dual-console* mode. The master controllers can be assigned in multiple

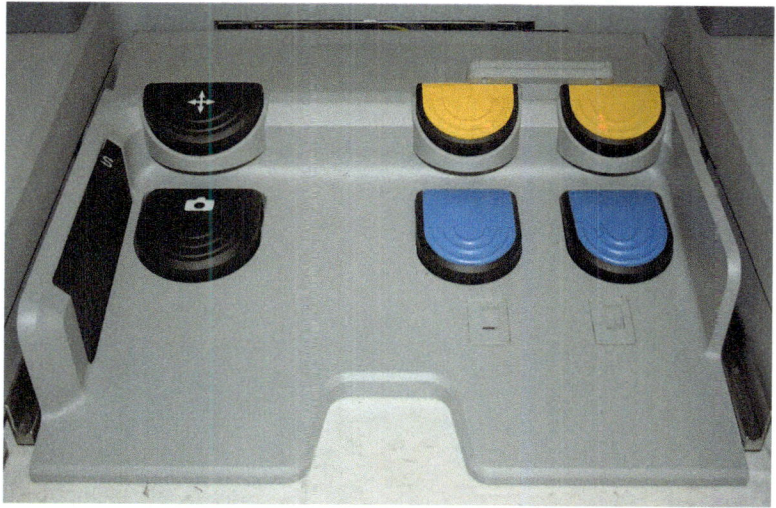

Fig. 2.7 The da Vinci® footswitch panel

ways to the two surgeons and can also be used for telestration for teaching purposes. The dual-console setup is particularly useful in a training situation.

The skill-based surgical *simulator* (Fig. 2.8) can be attached to the da Vinci® Si Surgical console. It contains a variety of exercises and scenarios specifically designed to give users the opportunity to improve their proficiency with the da Vinci console controls. This simulator was developed in collaboration with Mimic® Technologies. The Skills Simulator exercises range from basic to advanced and are designed to be relevant to surgeons from any specialty. The exercises are organized into training units and cover the most useful da Vinci actions including *EndoWrist®* manipulation, camera and clutching, fourth arm integration, and others.

2.2.2 The da Vinci® Components: The Patient Cart

The patient cart is the central patient-oriented component of the da Vinci Surgical System. It allows the camera and instruments to be introduced into the surgical field and provides a stable platform during the procedure. The major components of this part of the robotic system include setup joints, instruments arms, and a camera arm. These elements hold the EndoWrist instruments and the endoscope. The da Vinci® patient cart is equipped with a motor drive to allow for easy transport and precise positioning relative to the patient. The *motor drive* of the surgical cart is located in the back and includes a steering column, throttle, throttle-enable switch, and shift switches. It is designed to provide faster and easier docking and operating room configuration.

Fig. 2.8 The da Vinci® simulator

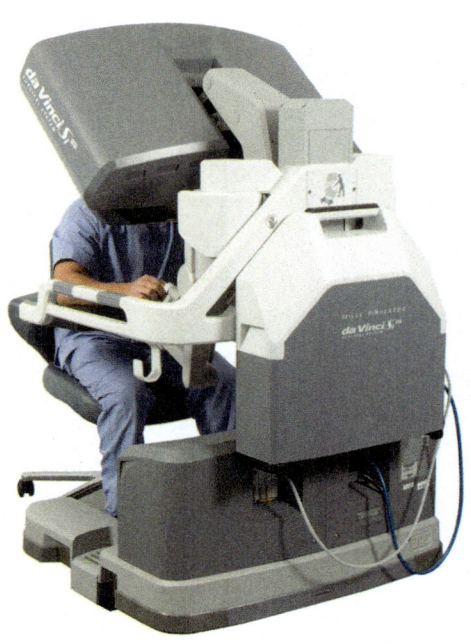

The *setup joints* of the da Vinci® patient cart allow for humanlike arm movements of the robotic arms. They are used to position the patient cart arms during sterile draping and to establish the remote center in the surgical field to maximize range of motion of the instruments. Clutch buttons at several locations allow the user to arrange and position the setup joints for preparation before the procedure and for rearrangement of the setup during surgery as needed. In order to maximize patient safety, any clutch button action at the surgical cart simultaneously suspends all telepresence activities from the surgical console.

The *instrument arms* (Fig. 2.9) of the surgical console provide the interface for the EndoWrist instruments and the *camera arm* provides the same function for the endoscope. Currently, there is no cross-functionality established between these two different types of robotic arms. All robotic arms are covered with sterile drapes and there are sterile adapters for the camera and the instruments. As previously described, all robotic arms are controlled remotely from the surgical console during the procedure. Installation, removal, and exchange of the camera as well as the instruments are performed by a bedside assistant.

The EndoWrist instruments (Fig. 2.10) are mounted onto the robotic arms for use during surgery. Their design allows for seven degrees of freedom and about 90° of articulation in the wrist. This provides the surgeon with a natural dexterity and full range of motion within a minimally invasive setting. The main characteristics of the robotic instruments include: an appropriate end effector for the specific surgical task (the tip), the wrist, a shaft (the "arm"), release levers to provide a mechanism

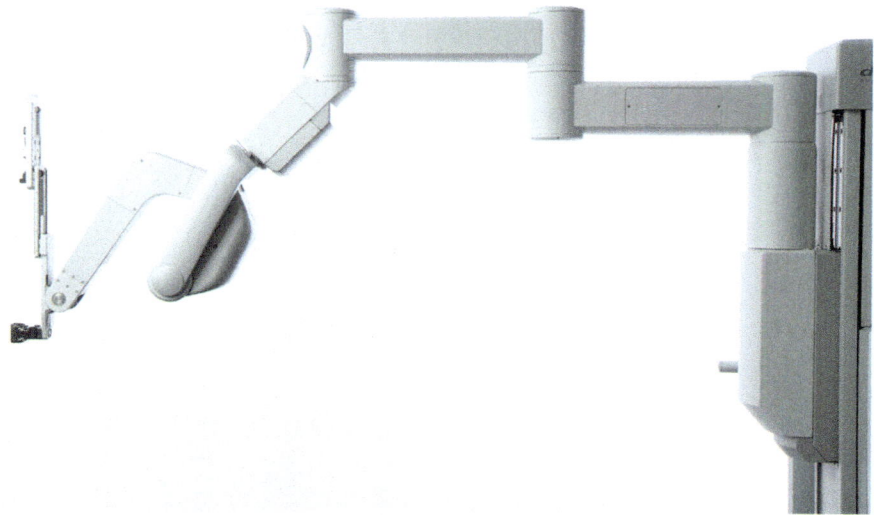

Fig. 2.9 The da Vinci® arm with setup joints

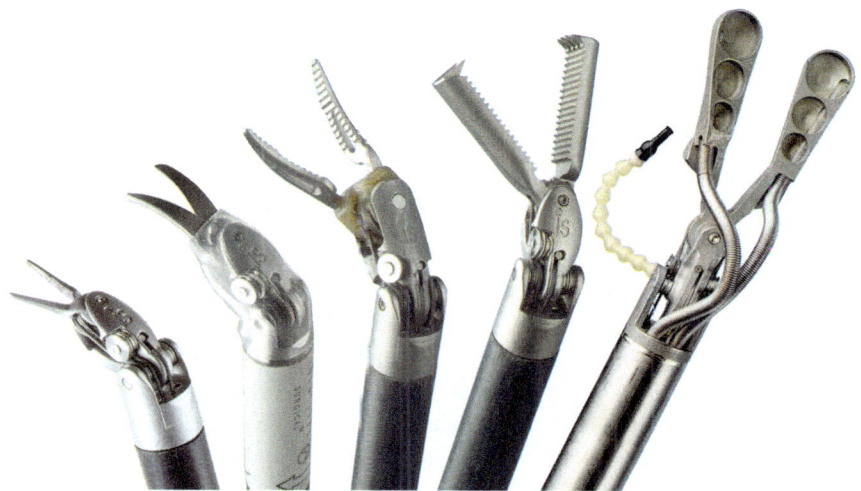

Fig. 2.10 The da Vinci® instruments

for instrument removal, and the instrument housing that engages with the sterile adapters of the instrument arm. A few of the da Vinci instruments are not articulated such as the Harmonic™ ACE and the single-site instruments, mainly for technical reasons.

Fig. 2.11 The da Vinci® single-site instruments

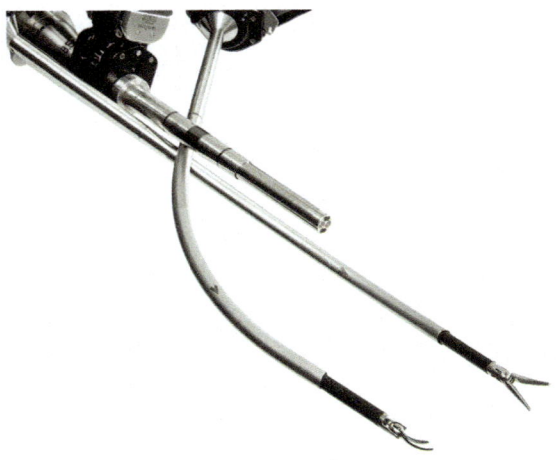

The da Vinci *Single-Site Instrumentation* kit (Fig. 2.11) contains material that has been specifically designed to enable robotic surgery using the da Vinci® Si System through a single skin incision of 2–2.5 cm. The kit includes a five-lumen port that provides access for an 8.5 mm endoscope, two curved single-site cannulae that cross at the level of the abdominal wall, an accessory port, and an insufflation adaptor. This design allows for optimized triangulation towards the targeted anatomy and provides an unobstructed view of the surgical field during single-site surgery. The curved architecture of the cannulae combined with crossing them at the remote center leads to a separation of the robotic arms outside the abdominal cavity. This avoids collisions and minimizes internal and external crowding. The robotic system automatically detects these specialized instruments and reassigns the surgeon's hands with the correct instrument to recreate intuitive control despite a crossed setup. The 5 mm robotic instruments are semirigid to accommodate the curved shape of the trocars and are not wristed. This instrument suite has been approved for cholecystectomy in the USA and is currently under investigation for several other procedures.

The *da Vinci® Si HD Vision System* can be used with either a 12 mm or an 8.5 mm endoscope. This rod lens scope is available in a straight configuration or a 30° angled tip. The illuminator that is located on the da Vinci surgical cart sends the light through the shaft of the endoscope via fiber optics and illuminates the surgical field. The video image is captured by the endoscope and is sent back through two separate channels to the camera head which contains two separate cameras, the camera control unit, and the illuminator. The endoscope also contains two separate optical chains and focusing elements. This results in a true and natural 3D image when displayed on two monitors to the left and right eyes of the surgeon.

2.2.3 The da Vinci® Components: The Vision Cart

The vision cart is home to the system's central processing and vision equipment. It contains a 24″ touchscreen monitor that allows the bedside assistant or other personnel to view the surgical images and to control central functions of the system. It also contains a microphone and speakers for two-way communication with the surgeon and has space for other equipment such as electrosurgical generators and insufflators. The vision cart also houses the da Vinci® Si core, which is the system's central connection point where all system, auxiliary equipment, and audiovisual connections are routed. The core of the da Vinci Surgical System is the location where all computed information is processed, including the motions of the instruments within the surgical field.

2.3 Conclusion

The current version of da Vinci® Surgical System is the product of a very successful, interdisciplinary effort. The developments from the first da Vinci® Standard over the S to the Si System coupled with growing adoption highlight the success of innovative robotic applications for minimally invasive laparoscopic surgery. Excellent clinical outcomes from various surgical specialties have been reported and will drive the further advance of this exciting technology to the benefit of many patients in the future.

Development of Robotic Systems

M.E. Hagen and M.J. Curet

3.1 Introduction

Descriptions of robots—portrayed as artificial helpers or companions—have been documented throughout human history. The ancient Greek god Hephaestus, for example, was said to have built automata of gold and silver to assist him in his forge. Other conceptions include automated "toys" such as a wooden, steam-propelled bird that was able to fly invented by Archytas of Tarentum about 420 BC and highly intelligent humanoids starring in movies such as I, Robot, the Terminator trilogy, or most recently in "Robot and Frank" (2012)—a movie picturing the intimate friendship between a retired burglar and his walking, talking helper who enables Frank to get back to his previous "occupation" despite progressing dementia.

The concept of using self-directed mechanical tools to supplant or augment human ability started to be developed into practical use in a wide range of applications beginning in the twentieth century. Today, robotics is a rapidly growing field as technical advances continue in various facets of everyday life. In the real world preprogrammed autonomous robots work well in automobile assembly and heavy industry where they function reliably on an assembly line with premeasured components. Therefore, it appears appealing to also use robotics in the field of surgery.

In that sense, the term "robotic surgery" conjures a variety of impressions at first hearing. The word "robot" suggests an autonomic system, like the droids of the "Star Wars" movies, which beep and whistle while pursuing their own highly technical agendas. Indeed, "The Empire Strikes Back" (1980) featured medical robots which treated Luke Skywalker for trauma and severe hypothermia and later

---

M.E. Hagen • M.J. Curet (✉)
Intuitive Surgical Incorporation, 1266 Kifer Road, Building 101,
Sunnyvale, CA 94086-5304, USA
e-mail: Myriam.Curet@intusurg.com

for the loss of his hand, all with apparent clinical competency and even a decent bedside manner in the absence of live practitioners.

However, a surgical operation is at this present stage far too unique, complex, and dynamic during its course to let a machine perform entirely without human control. Therefore, at this point in time, surgical robots are generally used for very specific surgical tasks such as reaming out a premeasured femur for a new hip implant, taking a biopsy from a site predetermined by radio imaging, or holding an endoscope during laparoscopic surgery. These robots are typically used by a surgeon to complete a particularly exacting segment of a more complex procedure and might be thought of as "smart power tools."

Still, robotic surgery has come a long way from the formation of the first research teams, early funding, and the market capitalization of a number of the products. The following chapter gives an overview on the origins and developments of currently available systems and examines the future of robotic surgery.

3.2 Development of Robotic Systems for Laparoscopic Surgery

While early attempts to perform endoscopic procedures date far back in time, the phenomenon of "modern" laparoscopy began when Prof. Semm from Kiel (Germany) reported his first laparoscopic appendectomy in 1981. Unfortunately, this innovation did not result in international acclaim for him, but rather disdain from his national peers who even suggested suspending him from clinical practice. However, in the years to follow, this new method of minimally invasive surgery on the abdomen progressively found its way into the operating theaters of Europe. In 1989, the first procedure videos were brought over the Atlantic and were presented at the annual meeting of the Society of American Gastrointestinal and Endoscopic Surgeons (SAGES, http://sageswiki.org/index.php?title=User:6365/SAGES_Milestones). In the following years, laparoscopic cholecystectomy became more widely adopted in the USA as the clinical benefits for the patients became clearer. However, it was also recognized that this new surgical method came with significant technical limitations including forced 2D visualization and poor ergonomics including limited articulation and the "fulcrum effect" that resulted in a significant rise of bile duct injuries, which is still observed until today and reported in the current literature [1]. Thus, manual laparoscopy presented an unmet technical need. These shortcomings significantly influenced the robotic surgery development as a means to improve the control of laparoscopic instruments.

With the emerging interest in applying robot technology to minimally invasive surgery, the second important influence appeared in the research arena of robotic surgery: the US military became interested in developing this approach to assist wounded soldiers on the battlefield [2]. After-action reports from the US Army Medical Corps showed that a significant number of serious trauma cases were liable to exsanguinate on the battlefield before reaching a surgical team for stabilization. Telesurgery was therefore envisioned as part of a medical evacuation system that would allow doctors to conduct remote trauma surgery on seriously wounded soldiers who were still on the battlefield or en route to a field hospital. The system was intended to fit inside a helicopter or ambulance and operate with the assistance of the infantry medics physically present with the patients. Eventually this plan was abandoned—mainly due to the changes in the accessibility of the developing battlefields—in favor of bringing advanced surgical aid stations closer to the battlefield. Still, the Defense Advanced Research Projects Agency (DARPA) made significant contributions to several groups in the nascent stages of robotic surgery.

Fundamental developments of endoscopic robotic surgery originated from transdisciplinary collaborations in Northern California's Silicon Valley, which is still home to the market leader in robotic surgery for minimally invasive abdominal and thoracic surgery—Intuitive Surgical Incorporation (Sunnyvale, CA, USA). The first efforts can be traced back to research during the 1980s that was performed by the National Aeronautics and Space Administration (NASA) Ames Research group located in the Silicon Valley. The team developed one of the first versions of a head-mounted display; it was used to transmit significant amounts of data that originated from NASA space missions to mission controllers. Around the same time, a company called VPL Research, Inc. developed the DataGlove—a wired glove that enabled interaction with virtual scenes—and the term "virtual reality" was coined. A later version of this technology called the "Power Glove" by Nintendo was promoted during the film "The Wizard" and the quote "I love the Power Glove. It's so bad!" became famous and is still a popular meme carried through the Internet. Some early conceptualizations of telepresence surgery combined these technologies into a visionary application in which data from the surgery was supposed to be displayed with the vision system while a robotic arm was to be controlled using the DataGlove. However, since NASA lacked robotic expertise, the Stanford Research Institute (SRI) with its own robotic knowledge and roboticist network was included in the efforts to develop a highly dexterous telemanipulator to enable complex microsurgery. SRI's system formed anastomoses in the hand of a patient while pursuing the original concept of telepresence. The emergence of laparoscopic surgery, combined with the US army's interest in macrosurgery to save exsanguinating soldiers off the battle field, influenced NASA, SRI, and Stanford University to divert their program towards a laparoscopic approach which was assisted by significant support from DARPA. Over the years to come, their efforts were very fruitful and the research ultimately produced a robotic endoscopic surgical system which was further developed and later commercialized by Intuitive Surgical Incorporation (Sunnyvale, CA, USA) as the da Vinci Surgical System®. For details on the further development and market launch of the da Vinci System®, please see the previous chapter.

While the da Vinci® Surgical System currently appears as the most significant robotic device for laparoscopy, the earliest commercial system for robotic laparoscopic surgery which was accepted by the surgical community was the automated endoscopic system for optimal positioning (AESOP). This system was developed by Computer Motion (Santa Barbara, CA, USA), a company that was founded with grants from NASA and the National Science Foundation's Small Business Innovation Research Program [3]. Later, the company also received funding from DARPA [3, 4]. With AESOP, the surgeon was able to control the motion of a laparoscopic camera attached to a robotic arm. AESOP eliminated the need for surgical staff to hold the camera in place during the procedure and it also allowed for a steadier view and more precise and consistent movements of the camera [5]. The AESOP arm used Computer Motion's voice recognition software to control the motion of the camera. Computer Motion's developments were based on the assumption that voice-controlled commands would be preferred in the operating room as opposed to alternatives such as eye tracking and head tracking, which control motion in response to movements of the surgeon's head. AESOP received approval by the Food and Drug Administration (FDA) in 1993 just shortly after its first human use [3].

After its initial success with AESOP, Computer Motion embarked on developing an entire robotic system with surgical manipulators based on three AESOP arms, of which two were assigned to host instruments and one for the endoscopic camera. This so-called ZEUS was originally designed for minimally invasive procedures such as beating heart and coronary artery bypass grafting [4]. Additionally, the system was also used for complex cardiac procedures such as mitral valve repairs. This clinical work starting in 1998 resulted in FDA approval in 2001. During early September of this year, the ZEUS had its clinical high water with Operation Lindberg—a transatlantic cholecystectomy with a surgeon working at the console in New York to control the patient-side manipulators in Strasbourg, France [6]. The ZEUS was—very similarly to the da Vinci Surgical System—a master-slave system with remote manipulators that were controlled from a surgical workstation. This system also offered tremor filtration and motion scaling. Computer Motion was acquired by Intuitive Surgical, Inc. in 2003. Shortly after, both AESOP and ZEUS were discontinued; a few AESOP systems can still be purchased at online medical equipment suppliers.

After the acquisition of Computer Motion, Intuitive Surgical remained to market the da Vinci® Surgical System. The da Vinci® System currently is offered with dual console capability, a wide range of specialized instruments including a single-site set, a surgical simulator, near-infrared imaging capabilities, and other advanced features such as surgical staplers and vessel sealing with wristed articulation. Upcoming additions include surgical staplers with wristed articulation and other advanced features. The system is successfully used in a wide range of abdominal and thoracic procedures [7–11]. Additionally, endoluminal operations such as transoral robotic surgery (TORS) have been developed [12]. Other emerging procedures include approaches through natural orifices such as the rectum in an attempt to further reduce the invasiveness of surgery [13].

3.3 Development and Commercialization of Robotic Systems for Other Fields of Surgery

Besides the research initiative that resulted in a capitalized system for minimally invasive surgery of the abdomen and the thoracic cavity, independent efforts in other fields of surgery were observed such as neurosurgery, orthopedics, and urology:

The first robotic surgeries on humans were conducted beginning in 1985 using a Unimation brand Programmable Universal Machine for Assembly (PUMA) model 200 to take intracranial neurological biopsies [14]. The PUMA 200 is essentially a servo-controlled arm, not too dissimilar from a human arm, with six degrees of freedom [15]. Researchers wished to develop a more precise method of directing biopsy sampling while minimizing damage to crucial structures in the brain. Two teams developed successful surgical setups using this robot, called the Neurosurgical Biopsy Robot and NeuroMate, respectively. The skull was first placed in a stereotactic frame and imaging was used to identify the relative position of the lesion to be biopsied. The robot was then able to precisely hold and move the biopsy needle towards the target, while the surgeon adjusted its path to avoid critical structures. These robots were used successfully on humans and NeuroMate has since been adapted for other neurosurgical tasks such as electrode placement, endoscopy, drug delivery, magnetic stimulation, and radiosurgery utilizing small radioactive emitters. Over time, the unwieldy stereotactic frame has been replaced by a smaller baseplate which is affixed to the skull prior to the surgery and then imaged to provide spatial references. The baseplate is then attached to the surgical system, which confirms its spatial model via ultrasound before the operation commences.

In 1991, robotics entered the field of urological surgery with the first successful human trial of Probot. Probot was designed to conduct transurethral resections of the prostate (TURPs), a long procedure in which it is difficult to position patients conveniently for human surgeons. Probot was an adapted PUMA 560 robot which was able to use eight degrees of freedom to swiftly core out a conical section from the prostate [16]. The only major adaptation added by the developers was a safety ring to circumscribe the potential range of motion of the arm. The result was a demonstrably faster and more precise procedure.

In 1992, human orthopedic surgery joined the robot ranks with a robotic system also based on the PUMA arm named ROBODOC which proved itself in animal trials first. One of the early developers of the system was a veterinary doctor and many dogs with fractured or dislocated hips were brought to the team for surgery. The clinical results of the rising number of total hip arthroplasties (THAs) demonstrated the difficulty of consistently and accurately reaming out the interior of the proximal femur to perfectly fit the tang of the implant. After implanting titanium fiducial pins into the condyles and greater trochanter, the femur is imaged and exposed and the neck is cut to remove the head before the bone is clamped to the robot at the lesser trochanter. The position of the fiduciaries is registered by the robot arm using a ball probe, which allows the computer to calculate a cutting path (using a virtual model created by earlier imaging) to create a cavity that will optimally support the implant [17]. The implantation procedure went much more smoothly with ROBODOC, although long-term outcome data is still lacking. Despite significant delays due to a lengthy approval process by the FDA, the ROBODOC was one of the first surgical robots to be commercialized.

The first purpose-built surgical robot was also for orthopedic surgery. Total knee replacements (TKRs) require similarly precise cuts to THAs, and Acrobot (Active

Constraint Robot) was developed to address this [18]. The surgeon first plans the procedure using a CT scan of the patient's knee to determine where the cuts will be made in the bone. After the knee is exposed via a medial parapatellar approach, the femur and tibia are clamped into place relative to the robot. Instead of using fiducials which must be implanted ahead of time, the surgeon "shows" the computer the bone's spatial positioning by directing a ball probe at the end of the manipulator arm over landmarks on the surface of the exposed bone. After registration to the imaging-derived model is confirmed and the patellar cuts are performed manually, the tibial and femoral cuts are performed using the robot. Although the robot controls the path of the cutting tool, the surgeon controls the force and speed of the cut by means of direct haptic feedback.

A similar approach for joint replacement is the more recent Robotic Arm Interactive Orthopedic System (RIO) by MAKO Surgical Corp. (Fort Lauderdale, FL, USA), an arm system which is intended for orthopedic procedures such as minimally invasive knee resurfacing and ultraprecise hip arthroplasty. MAKO was founded in 2004 and markets a family of implants together with the abovementioned systems for knee and hip replacements. The company currently claims to be protected by an intellectual property portfolio including more than 300 US and foreign, owned and licensed, patents and patent applications. The system enables the orthopedic surgeon to achieve reproducible precision for the patients. MAKOplasty® Partial Knee Resurfacing is a minimally invasive method for knee resurfacing designed to relieve pain and restore range of motion for adults living with early to mid-stage osteoarthritis that has not progressed to all three compartments of the knee [19, 20]. MAKOplasty® Total Hip Arthroplasty is a newer version of the RIO® robotic arm application for total hip replacement.

In 1987, CyberKnife was developed, an interventional radiological robot designed to allow a radiation oncologist to precisely target lesions with multiple small bursts of radiation intersecting the target from different angles, allowing minimal radiation exposure to healthy tissue while maximizing the cumulative dose applied to the lesion [21, 22]. Because the interior of the human body is a dynamic environment, CyberKnife updates its spatial registration prior to each dose using fluoroscopic imaging and predictive software to track and anticipate respiratory motion.

One of the latest surgical robots to be introduced is in the field of cardiac surgery. The CardioARM robot utilizes a slim snakelike manipulator which is able to slip into the thoracic cavity by means of a simple subxiphoid approach, obviating the need for thoracotomy [23]. It is also being considered for use in natural orifice transluminal endoscopic surgery (NOTES). Robots have also proven useful in controlling cardiac catheters. The Sensei system made by Hansen Medical utilizes a master-slave setup to allow remote control of a fluoroscopically guided catheter, preventing overexposure to radiation by the cardiologist. The more advanced Niobe system made by Stereotaxis guides the ferrous tip of the catheter through the major vessels and the heart using a magnetic field [24]. The Niobe computer is able to integrate real-time imaging data to produce 3D magnetic vectors to move and orient the catheter throughout the procedure as directed by the cardiologist. A similar system is also being developed to control intraluminal self-contained systems for gastrointestinal applications, which need not be attached to a base station—essentially a pill camera that can be driven remotely.

3.4 Future Systems for Laparoscopic Surgery

Besides concrete technical advantages of the currently available robotic systems such as the da Vinci® Surgical System, a prominent and promising feature of robotics derives from the fact that they are information-based systems. Therefore, they open the door for interfacing and integrating with many of the other technologies that are currently used in or around the field of surgery. These opportunities include the superimposition of preoperative imaging or the fusion of such data with the surgical video to allow a more precise dissection. These preoperative data sets will at some point in time allow preoperative planning and rehearsing of the surgical procedure. With further technical advance towards solutions around soft tissue deformation, it is imaginable that robotic procedures may be virtually "preperformed" by the surgeon with the help of preoperative imaging to determine the best approach. The robotic system is able to later perform the saved procedure on the real patient in a fraction of the time, minimizing time spent under the knife. Additionally, robotics has great potential in the fields of long-distance surgery and remote training of surgeons.

While the da Vinci Surgical System is currently the system for laparoscopic surgery and the system will certainly be continuously enhanced, other systems are under development and might surface into the clinical arena in the future. Some have been presented at conferences or information is available through the public domain:

Amongst them is an effort by the German Aerospace (DLR), whose Institute of Robotics and Mechatronics developed a versatile robotic arm for surgical applications. This MIRO system currently exists in the second generation. It is very similar in its proportions to a human arm, with a weight of about 10 kg. The robotic arms are directly installed to the operating table and controlled remotely. Targeted procedures range from orthopedics and laser surgery to a multi-robot setup for laparoscopy. This versatile approach enabled by the design of the system itself and the flexibility of the robotic control architecture is further supported by a wide range of instruments. The DLR group won several prizes with the design of the MIRO. However, until now there have been no reports of the application of this system on human patients.

Another project that is currently under development is the Amadeus system by Titan Medical in Toronto, Canada. The company's webpage reveals some information about their system: similar to the da Vinci Surgical System, the Amadeus appears to be a master-slave system with a surgeon's console that interfaces with a robotic platform. It includes a 3D vision system and interactive instruments with a setup for single-site as well as multiport capabilities. The instrument shafts are described to be flexible with multiple degrees of freedom. In addition, the description includes force feedback for detection of tissue-level forces. The claimed benefits of the system include higher dexterity and natural control of instruments with a flexible port access allowing multi-quadrant abdominal procedures.

ARAKNES (Array of Robots Augmenting the Kinematics of Endoluminal Surgery) is a project that is heavily co-funded by the European Commission within the Seventh Framework Program. This project brings together multiple academic institutes as well as corporations from Europe. The project is based on the concept of transferring the technology of bimanual laparoscopy to an endoluminal approach in an attempt to reduce surgical trauma and to enhance patient-oriented outcomes. The aim of this team effort is to design a system that results in bimanual, ambulatory, tethered, and visible scarless surgery by advancing the current endoscopic surgical procedures to include bimanual teleoperation equivalent to that of laparoscopic surgical robots.

In addition to these abovementioned projects that are currently known to exist, multiple other research teams are working on new solutions for the limitations of minimally invasive surgery. Several publications on concepts as well as very preliminary results can be found in the literature. Whether these new systems will appear on the market eventually or if they can add benefits to the currently available systems remains unclear at present. However, it is clear that robotics continues to grow within the surgical arena and that they will change the surgical landscape forever.

3.5 Conclusions

Despite these exciting developments in the flied of robotic surgery, this discipline is still in its infancy. While significant progress has been made up to the establishment of robotic surgery as the gold standard for certain procedures such as prostatectomy, many factors are still unknown and further obstacles have yet to be overcome.

Still, the current status of laparoscopic surgical robotics with 3D vision, eight degrees of freedom, a wide range of instruments, and important software features permits the clear statement that the technology has become superior when compared to manual laparoscopy. While the clinical value of robots in a variety of surgical applications has not yet been shown at the highest level of evidence, it appears justified to continue in the development and expansion of the field. However, many technical advances need to be made before the full potential of robotic surgery can be realized. Significantly more specialized mechanical instruments and more energy-directed tools need to be developed for use with surgical robotics. Integration of advanced diagnostic testing, ultrasonography, new imaging modalities, and more specialized equipment will further enhance the clinical variety of potential robotic applications.

As with the Hollywood robots of I, Robot and Terminator and their shiny metal friends, the future of robotic surgery is limited only by our imagination. The possibilities are endless and the future of robotics is the subject of intense research around the world. Robotics will profoundly enhance the practice of surgery and we are just beginning to see the revolutionary changes that it will bring.

References

1. Connor S, Garden OJ (2006) Bile duct injury in the era of laparoscopic cholecystectomy. Br J Surg 93:158–168
2. Satava RM (2002) Surgical robotics: the early chronicles: a personal historical perspective. Surg Laparosc Endosc Percutan Tech 12:6–16
3. Ewing DR, Pigazzi A, Wang Y, Ballantyne GH (2004) Robots in the operating room: the history. Semin Laparosc Surg 11:63–71
4. Satava RM (2003) Robotic surgery: from past to future: a personal journey. Surg Clin North Am 83:1491–1500, xii
5. Sackier JM, Wang Y (1994) Robotically assisted laparoscopic surgery. From concept to development. Surg Endosc 8:63–66
6. Marescaux J (2002) Code name: "Lindbergh operation". Ann Chir 127:2–4
7. Hagen ME, Pugin F, Chassot G, Huber O, Buchs N, Iranmanesh P, Morel P (2012) Reducing cost of surgery by avoiding complications: the model of robotic Roux-en-Y gastric bypass. Obes Surg 22(1):52–61
8. Baik SH (2008) Robotic colorectal surgery. Yonsei Med J 49:891–896
9. Newlin ME, Mikami DJ, Melvin SW (2004) Initial experience with the four-arm computer-enhanced telesurgery device in foregut surgery. J Laparoendosc Adv Surg Tech A 14:121–124
10. Choi GH, Choi SH, Kim SH, Hwang HK, Kang CM, Choi JS, Lee WJ (2012) Robotic liver resection: technique and results of 30 consecutive procedures. Surg Endosc 26:2247–2258
11. Augustin F, Bodner J, Wykypiel H, Schwinghammer C, Schmid T (2012) Perioperative results of robotic lung lobectomy: summary of literature. Surg Endosc 26:1190–1191
12. Genden EM, O'Malley BW Jr, Weinstein GS, Stucken CL, Selber JC, Rinaldo A, Hockstein NG, Ozer E, Mallet Y, Satava RM, Moore EJ, Silver CE, Ferlito A (2012) Transoral robotic surgery: role in the management of upper aerodigestive tract tumors. Head Neck 34:886–893
13. Hompes R, Rauh SM, Hagen ME, Mortensen NJ (2012) Preclinical cadaveric study of transanal endoscopic da Vinci(R) surgery. Br J Surg 99:1144–1148
14. Kwoh YS, Hou J, Jonckheere EA, Hayati S (1988) A robot with improved absolute positioning accuracy for CT guided stereotactic brain surgery. IEEE Trans Biomed Eng 35:153–160
15. Benabid AL, Cinquin P, Lavalle S, Le Bas JF, Demongeot J, de Rougemont J (1987) Computer-driven robot for stereotactic surgery connected to CT scan and magnetic resonance imaging. Technological design and preliminary results. Appl Neurophysiol 50:153–154
16. Bann S, Khan M, Hernandez J, Munz Y, Moorthy K, Datta V, Rockall T, Darzi A (2003) Robotics in surgery. J Am Coll Surg 196:784–795
17. Paul HA, Bargar WL, Mittlestadt B, Musits B, Taylor RH, Kazanzides P, Zuhars J, Williamson B, Hanson W (1992) Development of a surgical robot for cementless total hip arthroplasty. Clin Orthop Relat Res 265:57–66
18. Jakopec M, Harris SJ, Rodriguez y Baena F, Gomes P, Cobb J, Davies BL (2001) The first clinical application of a "hands-on" robotic knee surgery system. Comput Aided Surg 6:329–339
19. Lonner JH, John TK, Conditt MA (2010) Robotic arm-assisted UKA improves tibial component alignment: a pilot study. Clin Orthop Relat Res 468:141–146
20. Conditt MA, Roche MW (2009) Minimally invasive robotic-arm-guided unicompartmental knee arthroplasty. J Bone Joint Surg Am 91(Suppl 1):63–68
21. Adler JR Jr, Chang SD, Murphy MJ, Doty J, Geis P, Hancock SL (1997) The Cyberknife: a frameless robotic system for radiosurgery. Stereotact Funct Neurosurg 69:124–128
22. Adler JR Jr, Murphy MJ, Chang SD, Hancock SL (1999) Image-guided robotic radiosurgery. Neurosurgery 44:1299–1306, Discussion 1306-7
23. Ota T, Degani A, Schwartzman D, Zubiate B, McGarvey J, Choset H, Zenati MA (2009) A highly articulated robotic surgical system for minimally invasive surgery. Ann Thorac Surg 87:1253–1256
24. Malcolme-Lawes L, Kanagaratnam P (2010) Robotic navigation and ablation. Minerva Cardioangiol 58:691–699

Robotic Surgery in Urology

Masaaki Tachibana and Kunihiko Yoshioka

Abbreviations

EBL   Estimate blood loss
PSM   Positive surgical margin
SD   Standard deviation

4.1 Introduction

Robotic urologic surgery, an exciting and new emerging frontier in the field of urology, has large potential to progress in the future. Niguen and Das [1] and Long et al. [2] well reviewed the potential benefits of the robotic surgery in urologic surgery. It is important that urologists should keep interest of the new technologies and understand their limitations and the possibility of incorporating them in day-to-day surgery. Advanced robotic surgery was first introduced into urology in 2000. The early studies showed the feasibility and safety of the da Vinci (Intuitive Surgical Inc., Sunnyvale, CA) telemanipulator assistance in radical prostatectomy [3–9], and the technique extended to pyelo-ureteric junction obstruction [10–14], radical cystectomy [15–20], and partial nephrectomy [21–24]. The miniature endowristed tools offer a potential advantage over standard laparoscopy in the accuracy of preparation and suturing. Other advantages are a three-dimensional vision system and unimpaired hand-eye coordination. Complex laparoscopic tasks are learned faster by using the robot, which may also explain the shorter learning curves required for radical prostatectomy than for traditional laparoscopic

M. Tachibana, M.D. (✉) • K. Yoshioka
Department of Urology, Tokyo Medical University, 6-1-1 Shinjuku, Shinjuku-ku, Tokyo 160-0022, Japan
e-mail: tachi@tokyo-med.ac.jp

procedure. This new technology has spread rapidly over the past 15 years. By 2006, approximately 60 % of radical prostatectomies in the USA was robot-assisted. Data on the functional and oncological outcomes are accruing but not yet conclusive. Therefore, controlled clinical trials and comparisons from various centers are further needed. Other important concerns are the cost and training implications. Future application may also allow integration of pre- and intraoperative imaging in the management of urological diseases. In the not too distant future, newer robotic instruments will be added to the armamentarium for performing different surgical procedures in urologic diseases.

There are a substantial number of reports on performing complex urological procedures with robotic assistance in humans that documented their safety, efficacy, and feasibility. Most of the recent reports pertaining to robotic surgery have been in the domain of localized prostate cancer (radical prostatectomy), bladder cancer (radical cystectomy and urinary diversion for muscle-invasive bladder cancer), kidney surgery (nephrectomy, donor nephrectomy, partial nephrectomy), pyelo-ureteric junction obstruction (pyeloplasty), and adrenal surgery.

This review article will describe feasibility, safety, efficiency, and reproducibility of the robotic surgery for the treatment of urologic disease and discuss the potential progression in the future.

4.2 Robot-Assisted Radical Prostatectomy

Patients diagnosed with clinically localized prostate cancer have more surgical treatment options than in the past. With regard to oncological outcomes and perioperative morbidity of prostate cancer, radical prostatectomy (RP) of localized prostate cancer has dramatically improved the results of surgical treatment [25].

It has two approaches such as open and minimally invasive prostatectomy. Open prostatectomy includes radical retropubic prostatectomy (RRP) and radical perineal prostatectomy (RPP).

In the 1990s, laparoscopic prostatectomy techniques were developed [26]. However, due to the technical difficulty of the procedure, this operation failed to attain widespread use until the advent of the da Vinci robotic interface by Intuitive Surgical Inc. [9].

Following the first reported robotic-assisted laparoscopic radical prostatectomy (RARP) by Binder et al. in 2001 [27], the procedure has been extensively used with encouraging results in the USA [28, 29].

Menon et al. standardized the RARP technique by describing the Vattikuti Institute Prostatectomy (VIP) [30, 31]. Since that time, the use of RARP has steadily increased [30, 31], and it is rapidly becoming the predominant form of surgical management for prostate cancer in the USA. In 2009, about 85 % of all radical prostatectomies in the USA were performed by assistance of the "da Vinci" surgical system [32, 33].

Hu et al. identified 14,727 men undergoing minimally invasive, perineal, and retropubic RP from 2003 to 2005 using nationally representative, employer-based

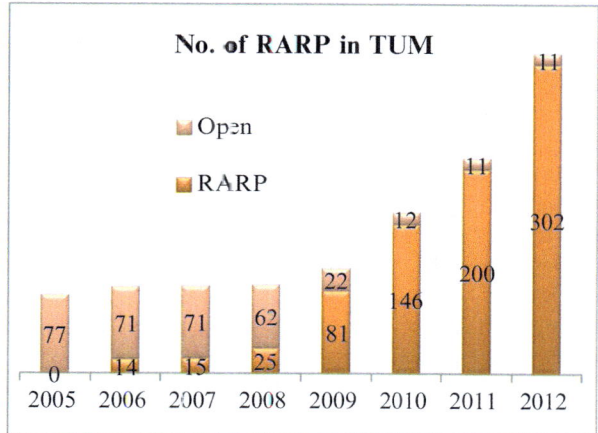

Fig. 4.1 Proportion of the open and robot-assisted radical prostatectomy at Tokyo Medical University Hospital. At the Tokyo Medical University Hospital, open prostatectomy was the main operative technique before 2006. In 2012, the number of RRP and RARP were 11 and 302 cases, respectively. Compared with 2006 and 2012, open surgery decreased from 83.5 % to 3.5 %, but RARP rapidly increased from 16.5 % to 96.5 %

administrative data. Use of the minimally invasive radical prostatectomy (laparoscopic and robotic-assisted) increased from 6.2 % in 2003 to 21.6 % in 2005, while use of the retropubic and/or perineal open radical prostatectomy (ORP) decreased from 86.6 % to 72.8 % and 5.2 % to 4.1 %, respectively [34]. Thus, laparoscopic radical prostatectomy (LRP) and robotic-assisted laparoscopic radical prostatectomy (RARP) rapidly comprise as a minimally invasive surgical technique to the treatment option for patients with localized prostate cancer.

At the Tokyo Medical University Hospital, open prostatectomy was the main operative technique before 2006. In 2012, the number of RRP and RARP were 11 and 302 cases, respectively. Compared with 2006 and 2012, open surgery decreased from 83.5 % to 3.5 %, but RARP rapidly increased from 16.5 % to 96.5 % (Fig. 4.1).

Multiple series of RARP are now mature enough to demonstrate their safety, efficiency, and reproducibility of the procedure, as well as oncological and functional outcomes comparable to RRP [29, 35, 36].

In general, it has been believed that pure LRP has a steep learning curve, but RARP is easier to learn and is now the surgical treatment choice in most centers of excellence in the USA. In 2007, it was estimated that approximately 63 % of RPs for localized prostate cancer were performed using the robot-assisted approach, 36 % by an open approach, and less than 1 % by the pure laparoscopic technique [35, 37]. There is now a significant number of literatures comparing prostate cancer outcomes after RRP, LRP, and RALP [29, 38].

Thus, robot-assisted radical prostatectomy (RARP) is rapidly gaining acceptance in the urologic surgery as a safe and efficacious treatment option for localized prostate cancer with comparable oncological and functional outcomes as open and laparoscopic counterparts [39]. RARP seems to have overtaken retropubic radical prostatectomy (RRP) as the treatment of choice due to patient preference for minimally invasive surgical options [3].

RARP has come a long way since the first large series appeared in the literature [4], and a recent analysis by Menon et al. found that RARP provided acceptable rates of biochemical recurrence rates (BCR) at 5 years for clinically localized prostate cancer [4]. This study was especially promising as it included a large cohort of patients for analysis and demonstrated that when an experienced and well-trained surgeon performs RARP, adequate long-term oncological efficacy will be obtained [4].

Newly emerging evidence reinforces this point, with RARP having lower rates of positive surgical margins (PSM) than RRP and LRP [3].

In one of the largest studies to date, Menon et al. [5] found that their VIP technique achieved comparable oncological outcomes to conventional nerve-sparing modalities and their results offered that 84 % of patients achieved total urinary control at a mean 12-month follow-up, with a further 8 % using liners for reassurance purposes.

Furthermore, the VIP technique utilized the increased dexterity of the robot's wristed instruments and high-magnification 3D view to ensure preservation of the lateral prostatic fascia, which conferred better erectile function postoperatively as compared to conventional open surgery [4]. The aforementioned results were corraborated in a meta-analysis from various high-volume centers, which revealed that RARP had quicken return of urinary continence and improved sexual function postoperatively than open and laparoscopic modalities [15, 35, 36]. Patel et al. recently reported that the age of the patient had a significant factor on potency after RARP, with younger men having quicker return to sexual function at 6 weeks, 3, 6, and 12 months postoperatively [7].

Complication rates after RARP in a recent study of 2,500 patients were found to be 5.08 %, with the vast majority of complications being either Clavien grade I or II [6]. RARP also seemed to have decreased intraoperative estimated blood loss (EBL), risk of intraoperative transfusion, and anastomotic strictures in comparison with RRP [3]. Coupled with the fact that RARP seems to have a shorter learning curve than LRP [9], it appears that the use of robotic surgery in the realm of localized prostate cancer will reach ever greater heights.

4.2.1 Robotic-Assisted Laparoscopic Radical Prostatectomy: Initial 15 Cases in Japan

Unfortunately, introduction of the robotic surgery in Japan has been far behind from the USA and/or Europe. The clinical trial using da Vinci surgical system in Japan was started by two university hospitals in 2000. However, for some uncertain reason, further development has not been progressed.

Since August 2006, our department has been started the first clinical trial of the robot-assisted radical prostatectomy in Japan [40].

Two of the present surgeons received a designated two-day training course under the guidance of Prof. Vipul R. Patel at the Department of Urology, Ohio State University. This training and licensing center is accredited by Intuitive Surgical, Inc., and the two surgeons became the first Japanese urologists licensed for clinical use of the da Vinci surgical unit.

The two surgeons then underwent their educational training program. The program consisted of (a) image training delivered to the prospective operators daily over a period of 4 months with viewing of surgical videos from the standpoints of a console surgeon and of an assistant; (b) weekly dry lab training using a sham pelvic cavity model and the da Vinci robot to practice the vesico-urethral anastomosis and dorsal vein complex (DVC) processing and ligature; and (c) after the two operators had performed 12 RALPs, mentorship was obtained for several cases from an expert in the procedure.

Between August and December 2006, 15 RALPs were performed (Operator 1 performed 12 cases and Operator 2 performed 3 cases). The procedure was performed as described by Patel et al. [28]. The operative procedure was divided into five consecutive stages: (a) bladder takedown, (b) dissection of the endopelvic fascia and dorsal venous complex, (c) bladder neck and posterior dissection, (d) preservation and/or dissection of the neurovascular bundles, and (e) vesico-urethral anastomosis.

RALP was completed successfully in all patients without open conversion except for the first patient, in whom a restriction to a 2-h operation had been imposed by the Ethics Committee. For the 14 patients, the mean operative time was 322.1 min (setup time, 41.6 min; console time, 233.9 min) and the mean blood loss (including urine) was 392.5 mL. The mean console time and the mean blood loss (including urine) improved from 264.2 min and 462.3 mL for the first 11 cases to 151 min and 136.7 mL, respectively, for the last three cases [40].

When the times required to complete each stage of the operative procedure were analyzed, there was a progressive reduction in operative times for all operative stages, with increasing experience. All 14 patients had a favorable postoperative course. There were no intraoperative or early postoperative complications. The average duration of postoperative catheterization was 12 days. The mean duration of hospital stay was 16.3 days. This long hospital stay was explained by the unique Japanese medical insurance system and the patient's demand regarding what they did not prefer to discharge before removal of the urethral catheter.

Between August 2006 and December 2012, a total of 783 patients with localized prostate cancer underwent RARP by a total of seven surgeons at Tokyo Medical University Hospital [41]. Among these are the initial 200 consecutive cases which were operated by a single surgeon. Prospectively the perioperative data with regard to patient's demographics and perioperative outcomes including oncological and functional results were analyzed. In brief, bladder neck preserving procedure was attempted for all cases using two different approaches. The posterior rhabdosphincter reconstruction technique was carried out just prior to vesico-urethral anastomosis [42]. The urethral catheter was routinely removed on the sixth postoperative day after evaluating cystourethrography. PSMs were defined as the presence of cancer tissue on the inked surface of the specimen. Urinary continence was defined as 0 or 1 safety pad usage a day.

The surgeon had no experience for conventional laparoscopic surgery including LRP prior to starting RARP, though he had extensive experiences with ORP.

The average of total operative time was 190 min with EBL of 252 mL. A total of 36 complications were observed in 30 patients (15.0 %) with no mortality. Twenty-nine patients treated with neoadjuvant hormone therapy and patients with pathological T0 stage were excluded in evaluating PSM for accurate data interpretation.

Within the 200 patients, the results of the first 25 cases were compared with those of the remaining 175 cases, the first 50 with the remaining 150, the first 75 with the remaining 125, and so on. Similarly, the effect of surgeon volume on total operative time and EBL was assessed using linear regression and Spearman's rank-order correlation coefficient. We defined the maximum surgeon volume as significant sloping learning curve.

A significant association was not observed between surgeon volume and other variables (age, serum PSA level, clinical T stage, prostate volume, biopsy Gleason score, D'Amico's risk classification, pathological T stage, pathological Gleason sore and the rate of nerve-sparing procedure). The median follow-up period was 16 (mean 20 ± 1; range 4–61) months. In 96 patients (48.0 %), the nerve-sparing procedure was accomplished, comprised of 82 unilateral and 14 bilateral cases.

PSM was found in 40 patients (23.5 %) out of 170. PSM rates were 9.8 % for pT2 and 54.2 % for pT3. Among 40 patients with PSM, 25 patients (62.5 %) had biochemical reccurrence (BCR:PSA>0.2ng/ml) postoperatively, who were placed under active surveillance. Meanwhile, of 130 patients without PSM, 10 patients (7.7 %) experienced BCR.

A total of 36 complications were seen in 30 patients with no mortality.

No intraoperative complication was observed. Eight patients (4.0 %) temporarily required a prolonged placement of urethral catheter for 3–7 additional days because of acute urinary retention. Urinary leakage from the anastomosis was seen in five patients, all of which was successfully recovered by a conservative treatment with extended catheter placement for a week or two weeks. The mean hospitalized duration was 15 days. There was no association between the surgeon experience and the hospital stay. Correlations of total operative time, EBL, PSM rate, incontinence rate, and complication rate with surgeon volume were evaluated. The average total operative time was 190 min (range 129–413 min). The sloping learning curve for this surgeon showed that total operative time was decreased with accumulation of experience in initial 25 cases ($p < 0.001$). However, total operative time of next 175 cases was not correlated with surgeon volume ($p = 0.288$). The average EBL was 250 mL (range 0–1,000 mL), which was not correlated with accumulation of experience ($p = 0.811$, Table 4.1). PSM rate of the first 50 cases was significantly higher than that of next 150 cases (34.8 % vs. 19.4 %, respectively, $p = 0.035$). Although PSM rate of the patients with pathologically organ-confined disease (Stage T2) was not correlated with surgeon volume ($p = 0.321$), PSM rate with pathologically extracapsular extension disease (Stage T3) was significantly correlated with surgeon volume ($p = 0.029$). Complication rate was also correlated

Table 4.1 Learning curve and perioperative outcomes of robot-assisted laparoscopic radical prostatectomy in 200 initial Japanese cases by a single surgeon at Tokyo Medical University Hospital

Cases	EBL (mL, mean ± SD)	Operation time (min, mean ± SD)	Incontinence rates (%)	PSM (%)	Complication (%)
1–50	267.2 ± 186.3	233.3 ± 56.9	24	34	32
51–100	193.3 ± 163.1	185.6 ± 32.7	14	22	12
101–150	263.1 ± 239.3	173.3 ± 23.9	6	18	12
151–200	256.2 ± 210.5	183.1 ± 30.1	2	16	151–200
Overall	245.0 ± 204.0	191.3 ± 42.5	11.5	22.5	17.5

with surgeon volume. Complication rate of the first 50 patients was significantly higher than that of the remaining 150 patients ($p = 0.002$). Of 197 patients, 173 (87.8 %) and 175 (88.8 %) patients achieved continence at 6 and 12 months, respectively. Incontinence rate at 6 months was 26.0 %, 12.8 %, 6.0 % and 4.0 % of the first, the second, the third, and the forth 50 cases, respectively (Table 4.1). Incontinence rate at 6 months of the first 100 cases was significantly higher than that of the next 100 cases (19.6 % vs 5.0 %, respectively, $p = 0.002$). To acquire the stable skill for total operative time, PSM rate, complication rate, and incontinence rate, slope learning curves of 25, 50, 50, and 100 cases were required, respectively (Table 4.1) [41].

These results demonstrated that the functional and oncological results of RARP procedure seem to be very promising. The learning curve is shorter in RARP than in conventional LRP.

However, much longer follow-up of patients and larger prospective studies are necessary to ensure current results.

4.2.2 Double-Layered Posterior Rhabdosphincter Reconstruction on Early Recovery of Urinary Continence After Robot-Assisted Radical Prostatectomy

The usefulness of posterior rhabdosphincter reconstruction (PR) during robot-assisted radical prostatectomy (RARP) has still been controversial. We investigated the association of several factors, including the Rocco original double-layered PR, with early recovery of urinary continence after RARP [42].

Between August 2006 and April 2011, a single surgeon at Tokyo Medical University Hospital performed 206 RARPs. Of these 206 patients, 199 eligible patients were enrolled in this study. We retrospectively analyzed the correlation of several perioperative factors, including surgical techniques, with early recovery of urinary continence 1 month after catheter removal. Continence was defined as no use or the use of only one safety pad per day.

Univariate analysis showed that surgeon experience, lateral approach of bladder neck preservation, bladder neck reconstruction, anterior reconstruction, and the Rocco double-layered PR were significantly associated with early recovery of urinary continence 1 month after catheter removal. Preoperative prostate-specific antigen (PSA) level, body mass index, and attempted nerve-sparing (NS) procedures, however, were not significantly associated with early recovery of urinary continence. Multivariate logistic regression analysis showed that the Rocco PR and attempted NS were the only independent predictive factors of urinary continence recovery 1 month after catheter removal (odds ratio [OR], 15.01; 95 % confidence interval [CI], 3.413–66.67; $P=0.0003$ and OR, 2.248; 95 % CI, 1.048–4.975; $P=0.0402$, respectively). When we applied NS as well as the Rocco PR, the recovery rate of continence at 1 month after catheter removal was 85.3 %.

These data suggested that the Rocco double-layered PR and attempted NS and not surgeon experience were the significant independent predictive factors of early recovery of urinary continence after RARP. NS procedures positively influenced early recovery of urinary continence only when they were applied with the PR technique.

4.2.3 Predictors for PSMs After Robot-Assisted Radical Prostatectomy: A Single Surgeon's Series in Japan

The prognosis after RARP may be predicted using multiple well-defined preoperative and pathological risk factors.

Therefore, we try to identify preoperative factors for predicting PSM in Japanese patients who underwent RARP performed by a single surgeon [41].

Between August 2006 and September 2011, a cohort of 244 patients underwent RARP performed by a single surgeon. We assessed the preoperative factors including age, body mass index, PSA level, PSA density, clinical T stage, prostate volume, surgeon volume, number of positive cores, and percentage of positive cores with regard to PSM.

In the univariate analyses, serum PSA level, PSA density, and surgeon volume were significantly associated with PSM. In the multivariate analysis, PSA density (hazard ratio [HR], 3.13; 95 % confidence interval, 1.57–6.24; $p=0.001$) and surgeon volume (HR, 2.15; 95 % CI, 1.06–4.35; $p=0.034$) were independent predictive factors for PSM. Using these two independent factors, we divided the patients into four groups and calculated the predictive probability of PSM. The predictive probability for PSM in each group was well correlated with the rates at 10.8 % and 10.2 %, 19.8 % and 20.0 %, 26.4 % and 26.4 %, and 43.5 % and 43.3 %, respectively.

These results indicate that PSA density and surgeon volume are independent predictors of PSM after RARP. A combination of these two factors can provide useful information about risk of PSM.

4.2.4 Conclusions

The clinical incidence of prostate cancer continues to increase in the patient population, and urologists struggle to identify those patients who require intervention for their disease and to determine which treatment modality is best. Active surveillance, brachytherapy, external beam radiation therapy, and RP are the current options for prostate cancer treatment. For many patients with a long life expectancy, RP may remains the most effective approach with respect to both oncological success and maximization of quality of life.

RARP has become popular among surgeons because of ease of pelvic access, high-power magnification, minimal bleeding, and decreased blood transfusion rates during the operation. However, it has not yet become the firmly established standard of care because long-term outcomes have not yet to be established.

Therefore, further prospective, randomized studies comparing both surgical techniques will be necessary in order to draw more definitive conclusions [34].

4.3 Robot-Assisted Radical Cystectomy

The incidence of developing carcinoma of the bladder increases following age [43]. Open radical cystectomy (ORC) has proven highly effective for control of muscle-invasive bladder cancer. However the surgery is associated with substantial perioperative morbidity. Therefore, in older patients who will be candidates for radical surgical treatments, thus it is imperative that minimally invasive surgical techniques should be demanded.

Over the past decade, minimally invasive surgical procedures have emerged as viable alternatives to several types of open surgery.

More recently, studies have demonstrated the feasibility of minimally invasive surgical treatment of muscle-invasive bladder cancer.

Robot-assisted radical cystectomy (RARC) offers an attractive minimally invasive alternative to the current gold standard of ORC for invasive bladder cancer [15].

Robot-assisted radical cystectomy is steadily growing with a feasible learning curve in those experienced in robotic prostatectomy. Pelvic lymphadenectomy appears to provide adequate nodal yield in several studies. Urinary diversions are most commonly performed extracorporeally, but several centers are attempting intracorporeal techniques. Short-term perioperative outcomes appear acceptable, but oncological efficacy remains unknown [44].

Initial results from an ongoing randomized trial showed no significant difference in the rate of PSMs or number of lymph nodes evaluated with robot-assisted laparoscopic surgery versus open radical cystectomy [44]. Parekh and his colleagues reported more large number of results [45]. In respect to their report, robotic surgery was associated with 50 % less blood loss, more than a threefold increase in the proportion of patients who left the hospital within 5 days, and a 20 % reduction in the rate of transfusion in the first 47 randomized patients. They also concluded that their results suggest no significant differences in surrogates of oncological efficacy and robotic-assisted laparoscopic radical cystectomy demonstrates potential benefits of decreased EBL and decreased hospital stay compared to open radical cystectomy. These results need to be evaluated in a larger multicenter, prospective and randomized clinical trial.

However, most of the favorable data for robotic-assisted radical cystectomy (RARC) has come from retrospective studies. The only prospective comparison suggested equivalence between RARC and open cystectomy with respect to pathologic outcomes and suggested potential advantages for RARC in terms of perioperative morbidity [20].

Therefore, Parekh and co-authors [45] acknowledged the need to validate the results in larger studies, and toward that end, he and his colleagues launched a phase III, multicenter trial to compare RARC and open radical cystectomy. They also indicated that they are assessing data on quality of life, activities of daily living, handgrip strength, and mobility data for all patients who have completed current analysis.

Robotic-assisted surgery for invasive bladder cancer caused less bleeding and allowed patients to return home sooner with no difference in oncological outcomes compared with conventional surgery. Pruthi et al. [19] reported in a small pilot study published in the Journal of Urology. The investigators reported that "initial results from an ongoing randomized trial showed no significant difference in the rate of PSMs or number of lymph nodes evaluated with robot-assisted laparoscopic surgery versus open radical cystectomy."

The interest generated since the initial description of RARC has been immense and larger case series are now appearing in the literature [46, 47]. Pruthi et al. [19] reported their initial experience with 100 patients who underwent RARC and found that there were no PSMs and that the mean hospital stay was 4.9 days, with mean bowel movement being at 2.8 days. Also, Menon et al. reported that the complication rate appeared to be 36 %, with 8 % of these being Clavien grade III or higher [5]. Nit et al. reported the first prospective randomized trial of ORC versus RARC in 41 patients and found that there was no significant difference in postoperative complication rate (33 % RARC vs. 50 % ORC; $P = 0.279$) and mean hospital stay (5.1 days RARC vs. 6.0 days ORC; $P = 0.239$) [20]. The investigators reported that RARC had a longer operative time than ORC (4.2 vs. 3.5 h; $P < 0.001$), but that there was less intraoperative EBL associated with RARC (258 vs. 575 mL; $P < 0.001$). More large series of the study [47], the incidence and predictors of PSMs in patients who underwent robot-assisted radical cystectomy for bladder cancer were evaluated using the International Robotic Cystectomy Consortium database; the authors identified 513 patients who underwent robot-assisted radical cystectomy, as done by a total of 22 surgeons at 15 institutions from 2003 to 2009. After stratification by age group, gender, pathological T stage, nodal status, sequential case number, and institutional volume, logistic regression was used to correlate variables with the likelihood of a PSM. Of the 513 patients 35 (6.8 %) had a PSM. Increasing 10-year age group, lymph node positivity and higher pathological T stage were significantly associated with an increased likelihood of a positive margin ($p = 0.010$, <0.001 and

$p < 0.001$, respectively). Gender, sequential case number, and institutional volume were not significantly associated with margin positivity. The rate of margin positive disease at cystectomy was 1.5 % for pT2 or less, 8.8 % for pT3, and 39 % for pT4 disease. Therefore, they concluded that PSM rates at robot-assisted radical cystectomy for advanced bladder cancer were similar to those in open cystectomy series in a large, multi-institutional, prospective cohort. Sequential case number, a surrogate for the learning curve, and institutional volume were not significantly associated with positive margins at robot-assisted radical cystectomy.

RARC also appeared to confer quicker time to bowel movement and time to flatus with less use of narcotic analgesics for pain relief [20]. This landmark study used a prospective randomized clinical trial to demonstrate that RARC was not inferior in comparison to ORC and matched up favorably with respect to various intraoperative and postoperative outcomes [20]. While there is still much work that needs to be done to assess long-term oncological outcomes, RARC is an evolving technique that affords patients and physicians alike an efficacious minimally invasive treatment option in the treatment of bladder cancer.

These results suggests that robotic-assisted surgery for invasive bladder cancer seems to be caused less bleeding, and allowed patients to return home shorter with no difference in oncological outcomes when compared with conventional surgical procedure. Those previously reported data suggest that "initial results from an ongoing randomized trial showed no significant difference in the rate of PSMs or number of lymph nodes evaluated with robot-assisted laparoscopic surgery versus open radical cystectomy."

Moreover, robot-assisted radical cystectomy with urinary diversion appears to be growing steadily in academic institutions. However, long-term data regarding oncological efficacy remain lacking but perioperative outcomes appear favorable.

Thus, RARC may reduce morbidity after cystectomy. Descriptions of the surgical techniques of RARC with intracorporeal orthotopic neobladder or ileal conduit are sparse, and oncological and functional outcome data have not been reported [47]. The authors concluded that RARC with totally intracorporeal urinary diversion is technically feasible with good intermediate-term oncological results. However, their results is a nonrandomized study including a limited number of patients with a restricted follow-up time; therefore precautions must be considered when interpreting the outcomes.

Between 2008 and 2011, 26 bladder cancer patients underwent radical cystectomy in our hospital (Tokyo Medical University Hospital), 11 robotically and 15 by open procedure. We prospectively collected perioperative and pathological data for these 26 patients and retrospectively compared these two different surgical procedures [48].

Eleven cases of RARC which performed at Tokyo Medical University Hospital were summarized in Table 4.2. Also, comparative perioperative and pathological results were shown in Table 4.3.

The RARC cohort had a significant decrease in both EBL (656.9 vs. 1788.7 mL, $P = 0.0015$) and allogeneic transfusion requirement (0 vs. 40 %, $P = 0.0237$). The total operative time was almost the same ($P = 0.2306$), but increased duration

Table 4.2 Summary of the surgical results which performed at Tokyo Medical University Hospital

Case	Diversion	Total of time (min)	Consol time (min)	Time for LN dissection (min)	Time for diversion (min)	EBL (cc)	Complications
1	Ileal conduit	437	215	40	147	717	No
2	Neobladder	345	123		305	772	Transfusion
3	Ileal conduit	409	140	10	230	485	No
4	Ileal conduit	377	189	50	137	258	No
5	Ileal conduit	313	155	20	136	241	No
6	Neobladder	508	160	22	257	1800	Transfusion
7	Ileal conduit	344	165	38	148	548	No
8	Neobladder	455	165	38	246	1010	Transfusion
9	Ileal conduit	453	186	24	250	281	No
10	Neobladder	477	196	25	265	475	No
11	Ileal conduit	418	140	37	72	189	No
Mean time (mins)		412.4	166.7	29.16	199.4		
Mean EBL (cc)						616	

Table 4.3 Perioperative outcomes of the robotic cohort (11 patients) and the open cohort (15 patients)

	RARC ($n=11$)	ORC ($n=15$)	P value
Mean estimated blood loss, mL (median)	656.9 (548)	1,788.7 (1465)	0.0015
Mean operative time, min (median)	408.5 (418)	363.5 (364)	0.2306
Time of bladder removal and lymphadenectomy, min (median)	157.6 (142)	117.6 (112)	0.0049
Intraoperative allogeneic transfusion, n (%)	0 (0)	6 (40.0)	0.0237
Time to resumption of a regular diet, days (median)	5.6 (5.0)	6.3 (6.0)	0.4190
Time of hospital stay, days (median)	40.2 (39)	37.0 (35.0)	0.4149
Incidence of intraoperative complication, n (%)	1 (9.1)	0 (0)	0.4231
Incidence of complication within 30 days, n (%)	6 (54.5)	11 (73.3)	0.4185
Clavien grade I	2	6	
Clavien grade II	4	4	
Clavien grade IIIa	0	1	
Clavien grade $\geq$ IIIb	0	0	

RARC robot-assisted radical cystectomy, *ORC* open radical cystectomy

of bladder removal and lymphadenectomy was observed in the RARC cohort ($P=0.0049$). Surgery-related complication rates within 30 days were not significantly different ($P=0.4185$). PSM was observed in three patients in the ORC cohort and in one patient in the RARC cohort ($P=0.4664$). The RARC cohort had a larger number of removed lymph nodes than the ORC cohort, and the difference was statistically significant (20.7 vs. 13.8, $P=0.0421$) (Table 4.3) [46].

Following our experience suggests that RARC is safe and yields acceptable outcomes in comparison with ORC for the treatment of bladder cancer if it is performed by a surgeon who has experience of over 60 cases of robot-assisted radical prostatectomy. This newly developed technique will gain acceptance as a minimally invasive surgery for muscle-invasive bladder cancer.

4.4 Robot-Assisted Partial Nephrectomy

The widespread use of radiological imaging (ultrasound, computed tomography, and magnetic resonance imaging) has resulted in a steady increase in the incidental diagnosis of small renal tumors. While open partial nephrectomy (OPN) remains the reference standard for the management of small renal tumors, laparoscopic partial nephrectomy (LPN) continues to evolve. The steep learning curve and technical demand of LPN make it challenging to establish this as a new procedure.

While OPN remains as the reference standard for these small tumors, LPN is now widely accepted as a feasible and safe alternative.

Oncological safety of this procedure has been demonstrated in published series reporting positive margin rates (0–3.6 %) and local recurrence rates (0–2 %)

comparable, if not better, to those reported in open series ranging from 0 % to 14 % [49] and 0 % to 10 % [50], respectively. Time has further evidenced the oncological safety of LPN, with reports from the largest series demonstrating a 5-year overall and cancer-specific survival rate of 86 % and 100 %, respectively [50].

Furthermore, with more than 1,600 published cases, clinical evidence has confirmed surgical outcomes comparable to those from open nephron-sparing surgery (NSS). Gill et al. [51] compared the surgical outcomes of 1,800 laparoscopic and open NSS procedures for single renal masses. On multivariate analysis, LPN was associated with a significantly shorter operative time, decreased operative blood loss, and shorter hospital stay. The chance of intraoperative complications was comparable in the two groups. However, LPN was associated with longer ischemia time ($P < 0.0001$). More importantly, although renal functional outcomes were similar in this study, and experimental as well as clinical evidence suggests a minimal impact of warm ischemia periods of up to 60 min, the potential impact of prolonged warm ischemia in the solitary kidney remains a crucial issue [51, 52].

Thus, NSS has become the definitive standard of care for treatment of most small renal tumors. LPN has been the traditional approach to minimally invasive NSS and has demonstrated decreased morbidity and equivalent long-term oncological outcomes compared to open surgery for T1 lesions. However, the technical and ergonomic challenge of laparoscopic suturing has limited the dissemination of LPN and has led to overuse of laparoscopic radical nephrectomy when NSS may be feasible.

Robotic technology has recently been applied to minimally invasive partial nephrectomy (MIPN) with the goal of facilitating renal function and reducing the learning curve (LC) for intracorporeal suturing.

Robot-assisted partial nephrectomy (RAPN) was first described in 2004 by Gettman et al. [21]. It has since enjoyed widespread adoption at many high-volume centers. Recent evidence suggests that RAPN offers equivalent oncological control to OPN and LPN while providing the additional benefit of shorter hospital stay, less intraoperative EBL, and shorter warm ischemia time (WIT) [53]. In an analysis of over 100 RAPN and LPN cases, no significant difference was found in the rate of focal positive margins between the two modalities [23]. While it may be too early to assess long-term oncological control in this relatively new surgical technique, early results from a series of 100 RAPN showed no tumor recurrence at 12 months [23]. Intraoperative EBL during partial nephrectomy has been shown to be an accurate predictor of early and late recovery of kidney function [54], and considering that 26 % of patients undergoing partial or radical nephrectomy have some degree of renal impairment preoperatively, [55] RAPN holds the promise of better long-term nephron preservation. Studies also show that RAPN generally provides shorter warm ischanic time (WIT) as compared to LPN [22, 23]. This seems to hold true even in cases that require calyceal repair, have complex renal tumors, or have multiple tumors [56]. New evidence reveals that RAPN has a relatively short learning curve with regard to parameters such as acceptable WIT and total operative time [57]. All the aforementioned advantages suggest, in our opinion, that RAPN will garner widespread acceptance as the minimally invasive treatment of choice for small renal tumors.

Furthermore, natural orifice translumenal endoscopic surgery (NOTES) for RAPN was recently assessed in a porcine model and while WIT was within acceptable standards, the great technical and surgical difficulty conferred with existing robotic instrumentation made the procedure especially laborious [58].

Domiguez-Escrig et al. well reviewed the technical consideration and an update of the technique for RAPN [59]. They concluded that the available data demonstrate feasibility as well as its functional and oncological safety of the RAPN. Robotic technology offers theoretical advantages over conventional LPN. However, the limited clinical evidence available has so far failed to demonstrate any clear advantage over conventional LPN.

4.5 Robot-Assisted Pyeloplasty

Robot-assisted pyeloplasty (RAP) provides a viable alternative to the current gold standard open approach for the treatment of ureteropelvic junction (UPJ) obstruction [1]. Gettman et al. reported one of the earlier comparisons of RAP with the laparoscopic approach and found that the robotic method was associated with less operating time [11]. Gupta and colleagues reported their initial experience with 86 patients and found that RAP was associated with a mean operative time of 121 min (mean anastomosis time of 47 min), mean EBL of 45 mL, and mean hospital stay of 2.5 days [10]. Most importantly, the success rate was found to be 97 % at a mean follow-up of 13.6 months [1]. A nonrandomized comparison of 30 patients who underwent RAP versus 30 patients who had laparoscopic pyeloplasty showed that RAP had decreased average operating time (98.54 vs. 142.25 min; $P < 0.001$), shorter suturing and antegrade stenting time (33.21 vs. 57.11 min; $P < 0.001$), and less dissection time (33.11 vs. 51 min; $P < 0.001$) [12]. RAP also provided less average EBL (40.36 vs. 101 mL; $P = 0.035$) and shorter mean hospital stay (2.5 vs. 5.5 days; $P = 0.036$) [12]. It is important to note that all 60 procedures in the above study were performed by a single surgeon who was an expert in both robotic and laparoscopic modalities and had passed the learning curve for both procedures. The authors thought that the robotic approach correlated more than laparoscopy with ease of dissection, efficiency in the tailoring of pelvic flaps, and elegance of suturing [12]. Recent reports have shown that RAP can be employed efficaciously in cases of complicated UPJ obstruction, which include horseshoe kidney, malrotated kidney, ectopic kidney, and giant hydronephrosis, to name a few [13]. Gupta et al. also described a transmesocolic approach to RAP for left UPJ obstruction in 24 patients, which had a perfect success rate at a mean 1-year follow-up with no repeat obstructions [14].

These data suggest that it is believe that RAP is an effective surgical technique for correction of UPJ obstruction.

4.6 Conclusion

Routine tele-surgery, smaller and more affordable systems, and the introduction of virtual reality, these developments have the potential to urological surgeons for improvement in their surgical results. Therefore, it is thought that these improvements bring the further spread of the robotic surgery in urological surgery. With the large potential advantages and latent qualities of robotic assistance in minimally invasive surgery over conventional surgery, robot-assisted surgeries may be developed to the next level and lead to a future revolution of the surgical techniques. Robot-assisted radical prostatectomy in the management of localized prostate cancer is one such example. The impact of robotics is therefore very promising.

References

1. Nguen MM, Das S (2004) The evolution of robotic urologic surgery. Urol Clin North Am 31(4):653–658
2. Long JA et al (2006) Use of robotics in laparoscopic urological surgery: state of the art. Prog Urol 16(1):3–11
3. Coelho RF, Rocco B, Patel MB, Orvieto MA, Chauhan S, Ficarra V et al (2010) Retropubic, laparoscopic, and robot-assisted radical prostatectomy: a critical review of outcomes reported by high-volume centers. J Endourol 24:2003–2015
4. Menon M, Hemal AK (2004) Vattikuti institute prostatectomy: a technique of robotic radical prostatectomy: experience in more than 1000 cases. J Endourol 18:611–619
5. Menon M, Bhandari M, Gupta N, Lane Z, Peabody JO, Rogers CG et al (2010) Biochemical recurrence following robot-assisted radical prostatectomy: analysis of 1384 patients with a median 5-year follow-up. Eur Urol 58:838–846
6. Menon M, Shrivastava A, Kaul S, Badani KK, Fumo M, Bhandari M et al (2007) Vattikuti institute prostatectomy: contemporary technique and analysis of results. Eur Urol 51:648–657
7. Patel VR, Coelho RF, Chauhan S, Orvieto MA, Palmer KJ, Rocco B et al (2010) Continence, potency and oncological outcomes after robotic-assisted radical prostatectomy: early trifecta results of a high-volume surgeon. BJU Int 106:696–702
8. Coelho RF, Palmer KJ, Rocco B, Moniz RR, Chauhan S, Orvieto MA et al (2010) Early complication rates in a single-surgeon series of 2500 robotic-assisted radical prostatectomies: report applying a standardized grading system. Eur Urol 57:945–952
9. Menon M, Shrivastava A, Tewari A, Sarle R, Hemal A, Peabody JO et al (2002) Laparoscopic and robot assisted radical prostatectomy: establishment of a structured program and preliminary analysis of outcomes. J Urol 168(3):945–949
10. Gupta NP, Nayyar R, Hemal AK, Mukherjee S, Kumar R, Dogra PN (2010) Outcome analysis of robotic pyeloplasty: a large single-centre experience. BJU Int 105:980–983
11. Gettman MT, Peschel R, Neururer R, Bartsch G (2002) A comparison of laparoscopic pyeloplasty performed with the daVinci robotic system versus standard laparoscopic techniques: initial clinical results. Eur Urol 42:453–457
12. Hemal AK, Mukherjee S, Singh K (2010) Laparoscopic pyeloplasty versus robotic pyeloplasty for ureteropelvic junction obstruction: a series of 60 cases performed by a single surgeon. Can J Urol 17:5012–5016
13. Nayyar R, Gupta NP, Hemal AK (2010) Robotic management of complicated ureteropelvic junction obstruction. World J Urol 28:599–602

14. Gupta NP, Mukherjee S, Nayyar R, Hemal AK, Kumar R (2009) Transmescolic robot-assisted pyeloplasty: single center experience. J Endourol 23:945–948
15. Richards KA, Hemal AK, Kader AK, Pettus JA (2010) Robot assisted laparoscopic pelvic lymphadenectomy at the time of radical cystectomy rivals that of open surgery: single institution report. Urology 76:1400–1404
16. Hemal AK, Abol-Enein H, Tewari A, Shrivastava A, Shoma AM, Ghoneim MA et al (2004) Robotic radical cystectomy and urinary diversion in the management of bladder cancer. Urol Clin North Am 31:719–729
17. Menon M, Hemal AK, Tewari A, Shrivastava A, Shoma AM, Abol-Ein H et al (2004) Robot-assisted radical cystectomy and urinary diversion in female patients: technique with preservation of the uterus and vagina. J Am Coll Surg 198:386–393
18. Menon M, Hemal AK, Tewari A, Shrivastava A, Shoma AM, El-Tabey NA et al (2003) Nerve-sparing robot-assisted radical cystoprostatectomy and urinary diversion. BJU Int 92:232–236
19. Pruthi RS, Nielsen ME, Nix J, Smith A, Schultz H, Wallen EM (2010) Robotic radical cystectomy for bladder cancer: surgical and pathological outcomes in 100 consecutive cases. J Urol 183:510–514
20. Nix J, Smith A, Kurpad R, Nielsen ME, Wallen EM, Pruthi RS (2010) Prospective randomized controlled trial of robotic versus open radical cystectomy for bladder cancer: perioperative and pathologic results. Eur Urol 57:196–201
21. Gettman MT, Blute ML, Chow GK, Neururer R, Bartsch G, Peschel R (2004) Robotic-assisted laparoscopic partial nephrectomy: technique and initial clinical experience with daVinci robotic system. Urology 64:914–918
22. Benway BM, Bhayani SB, Rogers CG, Dulabon LM, Patel MN, Lipkin M et al (2009) Robot assisted partial nephrectomy versus laparoscopic partial nephrectomy for renal tumors: a multi-institutional analysis of perioperative outcomes. J Urol 182:866–872
23. Wang AJ, Bhayani SB (2009) Robotic partial nephrectomy versus laparoscopic partial nephrectomy for renal cell carcinoma: single-surgeon analysis of >100 consecutive procedures. Urology 73:306–310
24. Scoll BJ, Uzzo RG, Chen DY, Boorjian SA, Kutikov A, Manley BJ et al (2010) Robot-assisted partial nephrectomy: a large single-institutional experience. Urology 75:1328–1334
25. Hammad FT (2008) Radical prostatectomy. Ann N Y Acad Sci 1138:267–277
26. Guillonneau B, Vallancien G (1999) Laparoscopic radical prostatectomy: initial experience and preliminary assessment after 65 operations. Prostate 39(1):71–75
27. Binder J, Kramer W (2001) Robotically-assisted laparoscopic radical prostatectomy. BJU Int 87(4):408–410
28. Patel VR, Tully AS, Holmes R et al (2005) Robotic radical prostatectomy in the community setting. The learning curve and beyond: initial 200 cases. J Urol 174:269–272
29. Ficarra E, Cavalleri S, Novara G et al (2007) Evidence from robot-assisted laparoscopic radical prostatectomy: a systematic review. Eur Urol 51:45–56
30. Hu JC, Wang Q, Pashos CL, Lipsitz SR, Keating NL (2008) Utilization and outcomes of minimally invasive radical prostatectomy. J Clin Oncol 26(14):2278–2284
31. Badani KK, Kaul S, Menon M (2007) Evolution of robotic radical prostatectomy: assessment after 2766 procedures. Cancer 110(9):1951–1958
32. John H (2008) Robotic laparoscopic radical prostatectomy: update 2008. Urologe A 47(3):291–298
33. Orvieto MA, Patel VR (2009) Evolution of robot-assisted radical prostatectomy. Scand J Surg 98(2):76–88
34. Hu JC, Hevelone ND, Ferreira MD et al (2008) Patterns of care for radical prostatectomy in the United States from 2003 to 2005. J Urol 180(5):1969–1974
35. Wagner A, Wei T, Dunn R et al (2007) Patient-reported outcomes after retropubic, laparoscopic, or robotic-assisted prostatectomy: results from a prospective, multi-center study. J Urol 177(Suppl 1):184

36. Krambeck AE, DiMarco DS, Rangel LJ et al (2009) Radical prostatectomy for prostatic adenocarcinoma: a matched comparison of open retropubic and robot-assisted techniques. BJU Int 103(4):448–453
37. Hakimi AA, Feder M, Ghavamian R (2007) Minimally invasive approaches to prostate cancer: a review of the current literature. Urol J 4(3):130–137
38. Hegarty NJ, Kaouk JH (2006) Radical prostatectomy: a comparison of open, laparoscopic and robot-assisted laparoscopic techniques. Can J Urol 13:56–61
39. Menon M (2011) Robot-assisted radical prostatectomy: is the dust settling? Eur Urol 59:7–9
40. Yoshioka K et al (2008) Robotic-assisted laparoscopic radical prostatectomy: initial 15 cases in Japan. J Robotic Surg 2:85–88
41. Hashimoto T et al (2013) Predictors for positive surgical margins after robot-assisted radical prostatectomy: a single surgeon's series in Japan. Int J Urol 20:873–878
42. Gondo T et al (2012) The powerful impact of double-layered posterior rhabdosphincter reconstruction on early recovery of urinary continence after robot-assisted radical prostatectomy. J Endourol 26:1159–1164
43. Jemal A, Siegel R, Ward E (2010) Cancer statistics, 2010. CA Cancer J Clin 60:277–300
44. Smith AB et al (2010) Current status of robot-assisted radical cystectomy. Curr Opin Urol 20:60–64
45. Parekh DJ et al (2013) Perioperative outcomes and oncologic efficacy from a pilot prospective randomized clinical trial of open versus robotic assisted radical cystectomy. J Urol 189(2):474–479
46. Hellenthal NJ et al (2010) Surgical margin status after robot assisted radical cystectomy: results from the international robotic cystectomy consortium. J Urol 184:87–91
47. Jonsson MN et al (2011) Robot-assisted radical cystectomy with intracorporeal urinary diversion in patients with transitional cell carcinoma of the bladder. Eur Urol 60:1066–1073
48. Gondo T et al (2012) Robotic versus open radical cystectomy: prospective comparison of perioperative and pathologic outcomes in Japan. Jpn J Clin Oncol 42:625–631
49. Yin M, Yang XQ, Li RB, Yang YQ, Yang M (2009) Retroperitoneal laparoscopic nephron-sparing surgery for renal tumors. Zhonghua Yi Xue Za Zhi 89:1983–1985
50. Lane BR, Gill IS (2007) 5-year outcomes of laparoscopic partial nephrectomy. J Urol 177:70–74
51. Gill IS, Lane BR, Blute ML, Babineau D, Colombo JR Jr, Frank I et al (2007) Comparison of 1,800 laparoscopic and open partial nephrectomies for single renal tumors. J Urol 178:41–46
52. Lane BR, Babineau D, Fergany AF, Kaouk JH, Gill IS (2008) Comparison of laparoscopic and open partial nephrectomy for tumor in a solitary kidney. J Urol 179:847–851
53. Brandina R, Aron M (2010) Laparoscopic partial nephrectomy: advances since 2005. Curr Opin Urol 20:111–118
54. Colli J, Martin B, Purcell M, Kim YI, Busby EJ (2011) Surgical factors affecting return of renal function after partial nephrectomy. Int Urol Nephrol 43(1):131–137
55. Huang WC, Levey AS, Serio AM, Snyder M, Vickers AJ, Raj GV et al (2006) Chronic kidney disease after nephrectomy in patients with renal cortical tumours: a retrospective cohort study. Lancet Oncol 7:735–740
56. Viprakasit DP, Altamar HO, Miller NL, Herrell SD (2010) Selective renal parenchymal clamping in robotic partial nephrectomy: initial experience. Urology 76:750–753
57. Haseebuddin M, Benway BM, Cabello JM, Bhayani SB (2010) Robot-assisted partial nephrectomy: evaluation of learning curve for an experienced renal surgeon. J Endourol 24:57–61
58. Haber GP, Crouzet S, Kamoi K, Berger A, Aron M, Goel R et al (2008) Robotic NOTES (natural orifice translumenal endoscopic surgery) in reconstructive urology: initial laboratory experience. Urology 71:996–1000
59. Dominguez-Escrig JL, Vasdev N, O'Riordon A, Soomro N (2011) Laparoscopic partial nephrectomy: technical considerations and an update. J Minim Access Surg 7(4):205–221

Robotic Gastrectomy for Gastric Cancer

Kazutaka Obama and Woo Jin Hyung

5.1 Introduction

Since the first application of laparoscopic surgery for gastric cancer was performed [1], laparoscopic gastrectomy has been accepted worldwide as a minimally invasive surgery (MIS) which provides reduced postoperative pain and faster recovery after operations [2]. As with open gastric cancer surgery, laparoscopic gastrectomy should be performed in accordance with the oncologic principles: radical lymphadenectomy according to the clinical stage of gastric cancer is required. Due to the technically demanding nature of conventional laparoscopic gastrectomy with D2 lymphadenectomy, the adoption of laparoscopic gastrectomy for advanced gastric cancer has been limited.

To overcome this technical difficulty, several experienced surgeons adopted the robotic gastrectomy for gastric cancer using the da Vinci® Surgical Systems (Intuitive Surgical, Sunnyvale, CA, USA) as a minimally invasive alternative to laparoscopic gastrectomy [3–9]. Robotic surgery system has technical advantages for operators, such as articulating instruments, an improved 3D magnified operative view, tremor filtering, and motion scaling. When compared to conventional laparoscopic gastrectomy, a robotic approach for gastric cancer surgery may facilitate potentially more precise and delicate lymph node dissection, thanks to these advantages. Since the first robotic gastrectomy for gastric cancer was reported in 2003 [10], several retrospective and small prospective studies have revealed that robotic gastrectomy is safe and feasible in terms of the known improved

---

K. Obama, M.D., Ph.D.
Department of Surgery, Kyoto City Hospital, Kyoto, Japan

W.J. Hyung, M.D., Ph.D. (✉)
Department of Surgery, Yonsei University College of Medicine, 50 Yonsei-ro Seodaemun-gu, Seoul 120-752, Republic of Korea
e-mail: wjhyung@yuhs.ac

postoperative outcomes of MIS such as reduced blood loss and shorter hospital stay [3–9]. However, because of the lack of randomized controlled trials demonstrating long-term outcomes, advantages of robotic approach from an oncologic point of view are still to be clarified.

In this chapter, we demonstrated procedural details of current practice of robotic surgery for gastric cancer. We also reviewed the literatures regarding robotic gastrectomy, as well as the possible advantages of robotic approach, especially for D2 lymphadenectomy.

5.2 Indications

The indications for robotic gastrectomy for gastric cancer are basically similar to those of the conventional laparoscopic gastrectomy. Patients with early gastric cancer without lymph node metastases ($cT_1N_0M_0$), which do not meet the criteria for endoscopic resection, are candidates for robotic gastrectomy with limited lymphadenectomy. cT_1 cancer with perigastric lymph node involvement and cT_{2-3} cancer with or without perigastric lymph node involvement are generally accepted indications for robotic gastrectomy with D2 lymphadenectomy. Basically, indications of surgery do not differ between robotic and laparoscopic approaches. Regarding locally advanced gastric cancer with obvious serosal invasion, direct invasion to adjacent organs, and/or bulky extraperigastric lymph node metastases, robotic surgery for these cancers is not generally accepted. However, robotic application for these cancers could be decided according to the surgeon's experience and expertise. In addition, robotic gastrectomy for those advanced gastric cancers should be carried out within the framework of clinical trials.

5.3 Operative Procedures

5.3.1 Operating Room Setup and Patient Positioning

5.3.1.1 Operating Room Setup
The operating room setup is shown in Fig. 5.1. The patient cart is positioned cephalad to the patient. The vision cart is located at the feet of the patient. The surgeon's console is placed where the operator is able to see and check the patient. The patient-side assistant is positioned to the left side of the patient. It is recommended for an assistant to have his/her own monitor on the opposite side of the patient. The scrub nurse is at the lower right side of the patient, which is on the opposite side of the patient-side assistant. Operating room configuration is usually dependent on the size of the room as well as the surgeon's preferences.

5.3.1.2 Patient Positioning
The patient is placed in the supine position with both arms alongside the body to prevent injury to the shoulders and arms. The operation table is tilted up to 15°

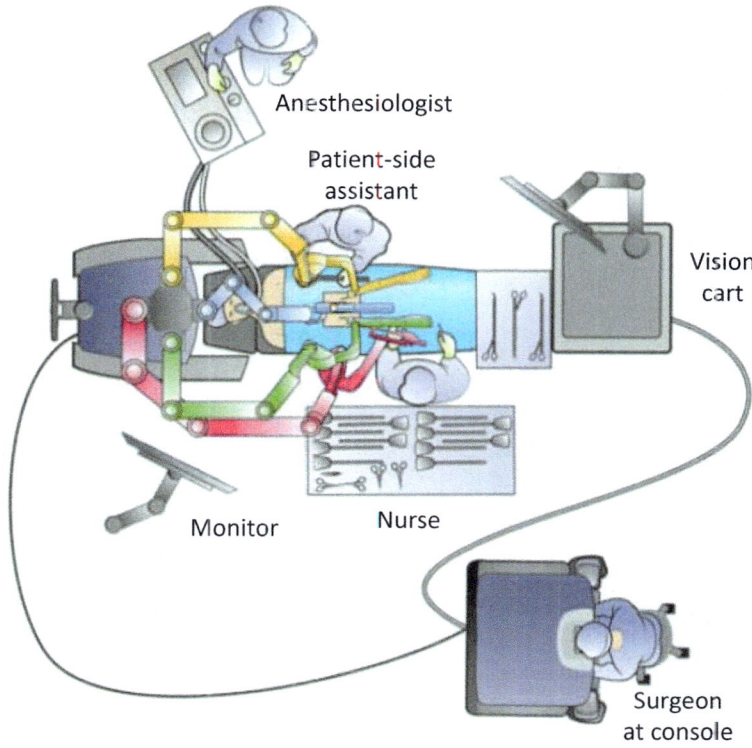

Fig. 5.1 Operating room setup. The assistant is positioned to the left side of the patient because the 3rd arm is deployed at the patient's right side and the assistant port is placed at the patient's left abdomen (cited from da Vinci Gastrectomy Procedure Guide)

reverse Trendelenburg position. In order to avoid any shifting of this position, the patient should be carefully secured with gel pads and a strap across the thigh.

5.3.2 Port Placement, Instrumentation, and Docking

5.3.2.1 Port Placement

Two 12 mm trocars (for a camera arm and an assistant) and three 8 mm cannulas (for robot arms) are used for robotic gastrectomy (Fig. 5.2). After the camera port is inserted through the infraumbilical vertical incision with the open method, pneumoperitoneum of 12 mmHg is achieved by insufflation of CO_2 gas. Then, surgeons assess the patient's abdominal cavity and check for optimal port sites under direct vision of the endoscope. The remaining four ports are placed thereafter. The left lower 12 mm port is used by the patient-side assistant. Practically, port placements sometimes require minor adjustments for the patient's body habitus. Notably, surgeons are recommended to maintain at least 8 cm between all ports. In

Fig. 5.2 Port placement and instruments. Note that distances between all ports should be maintained at least 8 cm. In order to obtain a good operative view during radical lymphadenectomy, surgeons should lift the camera cannula slightly anterior

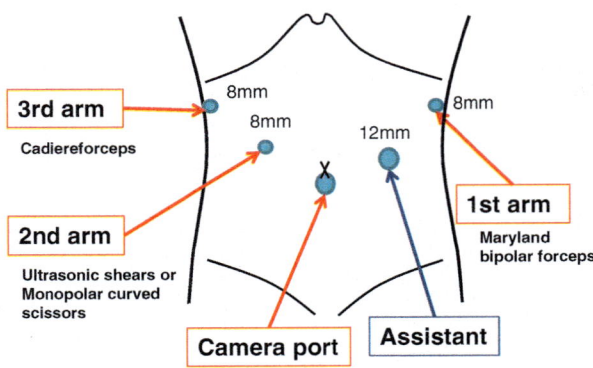

addition, both ports for the 1st arm (patient's left side) and the 3rd arm (patient's right side) should be placed as far lateral as possible.

5.3.2.2 Instrumentations

As shown in Fig. 5.2, the camera arm is docked to the infraumbilical port. The 1st arm holds the Maryland bipolar forceps. The 2nd and the 3rd arms hold the ultrasonic shears or the monopolar curved scissors and the Cadiere forceps, interchangeably. The 3rd arm is employed at the patient's right side because the 3rd arm should be at the opposite side of the 1st arm, which holds the Maryland forceps, for better countertraction.

5.3.2.3 Docking

After the adjustment of the camera arm setup joint toward the patient's left side (the side of the patient with just one instrument arm) and confirmation of the sweet spot, the patient cart is rolled in and positioned over the patient's head. Firstly, the camera arm is docked to the infraumbilical port. Then the three other robotic arms are connected to the ports. Surgeons should be careful to maximize spacing between the 2nd and 3rd arms by spreading these arms as far apart as possible.

5.3.3 Liver Retraction

Various methods of liver retraction have been described, such as the gauze-suspension method [11], suspension using Penrose drains [12], and retraction using Nathanson liver retractor [13]. Surgeons may adopt any retraction methods, as long as sufficient operative view is acquired. The gauze-suspension method is simple and not expensive and causes less damage to the liver than the Nathanson liver retractor [13]. Sufficient preparation of the operative field by appropriate liver retraction is necessary not only for accurate lymph node dissection, especially of the suprapancreatic area, but also for maximal use of instruments for dissection by eliminating the use of instrument for liver retraction.

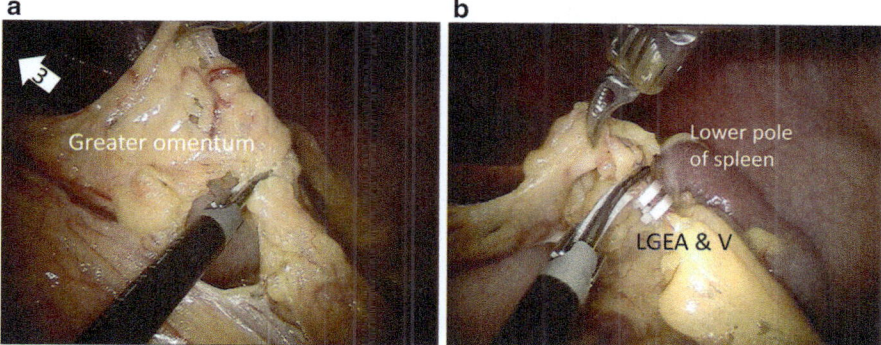

Fig. 5.3 Left side dissection of the greater curvature. (**a**) The greater omentum is divided at least 3 cm away from gastroepiploic vessels toward the lower pole of the spleen. *White arrow* indicates the direction of retraction by the 3rd arm. (**b**) The left gastroepiploic vessels (LGEA and V) are ligated by clips and divided

5.3.4 Distal Subtotal Gastrectomy with D2 Lymphadenectomy

5.3.4.1 Left Side Dissection

The safe division of the greater omentum is achieved by cephalad and ventral retraction of the stomach with the 3rd arm, which creates a draping of the greater omentum. After entering the lesser sac in the area of the mid-transverse colon, the greater omentum is divided at least 3 cm away from the gastroepiploic vessels toward the lower pole of the spleen using the ultrasonic shears (Fig. 5.3a).

The left gastroepiploic artery and vein are carefully identified, ligated, and divided at its root where lymph node #4sb is located (Fig. 5.3b). The omental branch should be preserved to preserve blood supply to the omentum. For better operative view, it is important to dissect the adhesions between the posterior wall of the stomach and the pancreas. Then, the soft tissue along the greater curvature of the stomach is cleared, which contains part of lymph node #4d, from the proximal resection margin to the short gastric vessel.

5.3.4.2 Infrapyloric Dissection and Duodenum Division

Complete dissection of the infrapyloric area containing lymph node #6 is one of the most difficult steps during radical lymphadenectomy for gastric cancer because of the complicated surgical anatomy of this area and easy bleeding. The transverse mesocolon should be appropriately taken down from the pancreatic head and the gastroepiploic pedicle. In this step, stable and appropriate retraction of the gastroepiploic pedicle by the 3rd arm provides better surgical view in the infrapyloric area. Before dissection of lymph node #6, it is important to have a better understanding of the surgical anatomy to release physiological adhesions between the transverse colon and the duodenum and between the pancreatic head

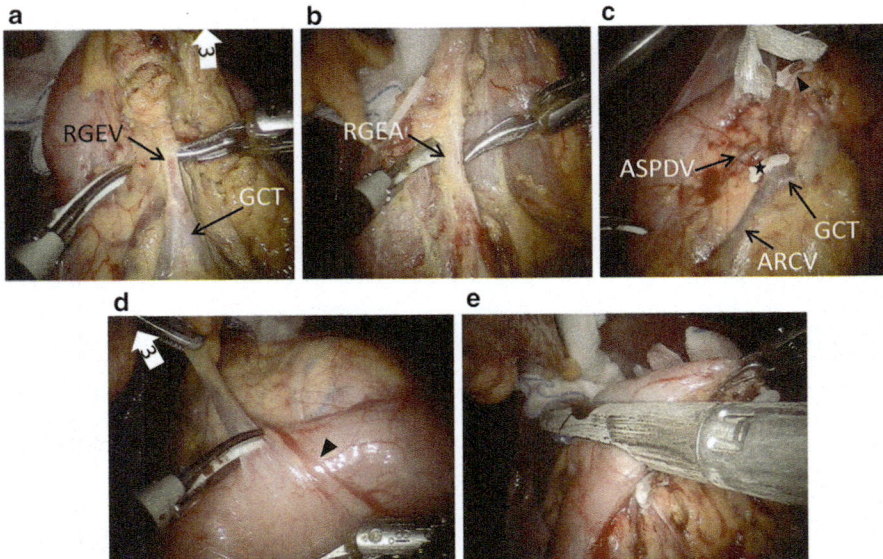

Fig. 5.4 Infrapyloric dissection and duodenum division. (**a**) The RGEV is identified, ligated by clips, and divided as it joins the ASPDV. *White arrow* indicates the direction of retraction by the 3rd arm. *GCT* gastrocolic trunk. (**b**) The right gastroepiploic artery (RGEA) is divided as it branches from the gastroduodenal artery (GDA). (**c**) After complete lymphadenectomy of lymph node #6. Note that lymph node #6 is bordered by the ASPDV, RGEV, and GCT. *ARCV*, accessory right colic vein; *arrow head*, stump of RGEA; *filled star*, stump of RGEV. (**d**) The supraduodenal area is dissected for duodenum division. Supraduodenal vessels are cut using ultrasonic shears (*arrow head*). (**e**) Duodenum division using an endoscopic linear stapler

and the posterior wall of the stomach. Note that lymph node #6 is bordered by the anterior superior pancreaticoduodenal vein (ASPDV), right gastroepiploic vein (RGEV), and gastrocolic trunk (GCT) (Fig. 5.4c).

RGEV is identified, ligated, and cut as it joins the ASPDV (Fig. 5.4a). Soft tissues anterior to the ASPDV and GCT should be cleared. On the left side of the RGEV, soft tissues superior to the level of GCT should be retrieved until the pancreatic parenchyma is exposed. On the right side of the REGV, soft tissues superior and anterior to the ASPDV should be dissected. Note that complete detachment of membranous tissues which directly cover the pancreatic parenchyma may cause potential leakage of pancreatic juice.

The right gastroepiploic artery (RGEA) is identified, ligated, and divided as it branches from the gastroduodenal artery (GDA) (Fig. 5.4b). Soft tissues around the root of RGEA should be dissected carefully to avoid injury of the small vessels and pancreatic parenchyma that is sometimes unexpectedly lifted up. The infrapyloric artery is usually encountered after division of RGEA. It may be ligated using clips, if necessary.

The attachments between the duodenum and the pancreatic head are released and the anterior side of the GDA is exposed. The direction of the ultrasonic shears of the 2nd arm fits the dissection of the GDA. After identification of the common hepatic artery (CHA), a 4" × 4" gauze is inserted anterior to the pancreatic head to facilitate the dissection of the supraduodenal area and to avoid injuries to the pancreatic head and major vessels such as the proper hepatic artery (PHA), CHA, and GDA.

The supraduodenal area is dissected for transection of the duodenum (Fig. 5.4d). Supraduodenal vessels are cut using ultrasonic shears. The duodenum is divided approximately 1–2 cm distal to the pylorus using an endoscopic linear stapler by the assistant at the patient's side (Fig. 5.4e).

5.3.4.3 Right Suprapancreatic Dissection

After transection of the duodenum, the stomach is retracted to the patient's left and ventral side to identify the right gastric vessels. Note that the hepatoduodenal ligament should be stretched using the Cadiere forceps of the 3rd arm with gauze for appropriate countertraction and better understanding of the surgical anatomy in this area. First, the anterolateral surface of the PHA is exposed to dissect adipose tissues around the root of RGA, which contains lymph node #5. Then, RGA is divided as it branches from PHA (Fig. 5.5a, b).

Through the whole process of suprapancreatic lymphadenectomy, it is an important concept to find the right plane between the major arteries and soft tissues containing target lymph nodes for safe and oncologically accurate surgery. Better operative view during dissection of lymph node #12a is obtained by stable retraction of the autonomic nerves along PHA by the Cadiere forceps to the right and caudal side (Fig. 5.5c). For complete D2 lymphadenectomy, soft tissues along the medial and posterior side of the PHA should be dissected to the left side of the portal vein (PV).

The anterior side of the CHA is exposed and soft tissues containing lymph node #8a are dissected from right to left until the bifurcation of the CHA and the splenic artery (SPA). Then, keeping the right plane between CHA and soft tissues, dissection of lymph node #8a proceeds to the cephalad direction of the CHA. To facilitate better operative view in this area, the assistant's retraction of nerves along the CHA dorsally and caudally is sometimes required (Fig. 5.5d).

The left gastric vein is identified and ligated using clips at the point where it joins the PV or splenic vein (SPV). Sometimes the left gastric vein drains anteriorly to SPV. Surgeons are encouraged to check the variation of the left gastric vein in advance by preoperative contrast-enhanced CT scan.

For retrieval of the right side of lymph node #9, it is required to dissect the soft tissue of the deep portion of the caudal side of the CHA until the celiac axis. Note that preservation of the nerve plexus of celiac axis is recommended in the case of "prophylactic" D2 lymphadenectomy. In general, dissection between the nerve sheath along the artery and soft tissues containing lymph nodes facilitates technically and oncologically safe radical lymphadenectomy.

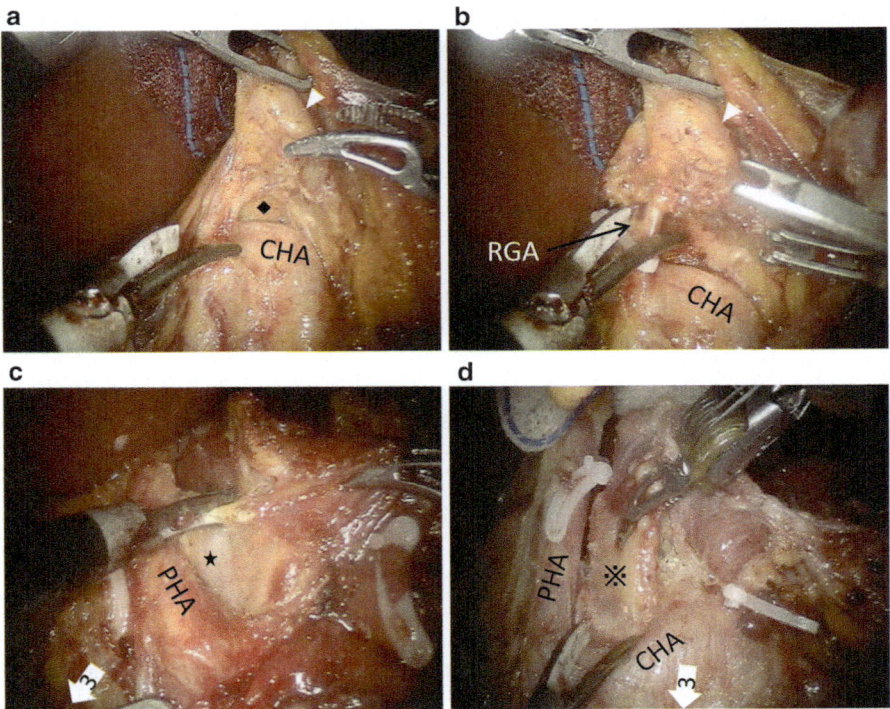

Fig. 5.5 Right suprapancreatic dissection. (**a**) Dissection of the avascular area (*diamond*) among the common hepatic artery (CHA), lymph node #8a (*arrow head*), and right gastric artery (RGA). (**b**) The RGA is ligated and cut at its root. *Arrow head* indicates lymph node #8a. (**c**) Dissection of lymph node #12a until the left side of the portal vein (*filled star*) is reached and exposed. Note that the autonomic nerve of the proper hepatic artery (PHA) is grabbed and retracted by the 3rd arm (*white arrow*) for better surgical view. (**d**) EndoWrist function enables surgeons to easily retrieve the deep dorsal portion of lymph nodes #8 and #9 (*reference mark*)

5.3.4.4 Dissection Around the Left Gastric Artery and Left Suprapancreatic Dissection

To completely dissect the soft tissues around the root of the left gastric artery (LGA) and celiac axis, the retroperitoneal attachments of the lesser curvature and the posterior stomach are divided from right to left side. The avascular area of the left side of the LGA and celiac axis is also exposed and dissected. Then, the LGA is exposed and securely ligated by clips at its origin (Fig. 5.6a).

The proximal portion of the SPA is exposed and soft tissues containing lymph node #11p are dissected along the SPA. The anterior and cephalad surfaces of the SPA should be exposed. Stable upward and left lateral retraction of the soft tissues containing lymph node #11p by robotic arm using articulating function allows surgeons to completely dissect the deep portion of lymph node 11p, which is usually one of the most technically demanding steps in conventional laparoscopic

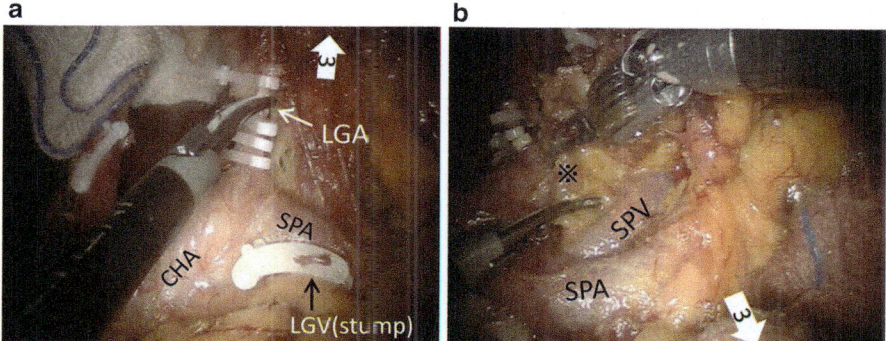

Fig. 5.6 Division of the left gastric artery (LGA) and left suprapancreatic dissection. (**a**) The soft tissues along the celiac axis, containing lymph nodes #7 and #9, are dissected and LGA is divided at its root. *CHA* common hepatic artery, *SPA* splenic artery, *LGV* left gastric vein. (**b**) Exposure of the anterior surface of the splenic vein (SPV) or dorsal side of the pancreatic parenchyma is desirable to completely dissect the deep dorsal portion of lymph node #11p (*reference mark*). The 3rd arm gently retracts the pancreas dorsally and caudally (*white arrow*) using gauze

gastrectomy. Exposure of the anterior surface of the SPV or dorsal side of the pancreatic parenchyma is desirable for complete retrieval of lymph node #11p (Fig. 5.6b). The distal boundary of lymph node #11p is delineated by the midpoint of the splenic vessels or the posterior gastric artery.

5.3.4.5 Lesser Curvature Dissection

After the gastrohepatic ligament is divided until the right side of the abdominal esophagus, soft tissues along the abdominal esophagus and the lesser curvature of the stomach are cleared until the proximal resection line to dissect lymph nodes #1 and #3 (Fig. 5.7a, b). During this step, the anterior and the posterior vagal nerve should be divided.

The stomach is then transected using two endoscopic linear staplers. Note that a sufficient proximal margin should be ensured.

5.3.5 Total Gastrectomy with D2 Lymphadenectomy

The options of D2 lymphadenectomy during total gastrectomy (TG) include spleen-preserving TG and TG with splenectomy. To avoid splenectomy-related postoperative complications, several surgeons have adopted spleen-preserving TG with D2 lymphadenectomy [14–16]. However, sufficient dissection of lymph node #10 located in the area of the splenic hilum is very difficult by conventional laparoscopic approach as will be described later. Robotic approach may allow surgeons to perform this technically difficult procedure more accurately with less

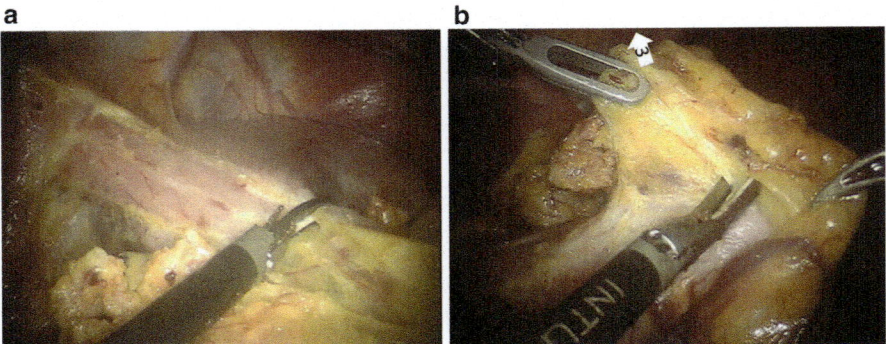

Fig. 5.7 Dissection of lymph nodes #1 and #3. (**a**) The soft tissues along the abdominal esophagus and the lesser curvature side of the stomach (lymph nodes #1 and #3a) are cleared until the proximal resection line from the anterior side. (**b**) The soft tissues are then dissected from the posterior side of the lesser curvature

bleeding without injuries to small vessels at the splenic hilum [17]. In this chapter, we focused on the spleen-preserving lymphadenectomy of station #10.

Dissection of the splenic hilum for lymphadenectomy of station #10 is performed after the division of the left gastroepiploic artery as it branches from the SPA. The branches of splenic vessels are exposed from lower to upper polar vessels. During this step, short gastric vessels are identified, ligated, and divided at its root (Fig. 5.8a). The soft tissues along the branches of splenic vessels should be completely retrieved using ultrasonic shears and Maryland bipolar forceps with articulating function (Fig. 5.8b). After division of the short gastric vessels, the esophagophrenic ligament is dissected and divided for enough mobilization of the abdominal esophagus to make an easier and tension-free anastomosis.

5.3.6 Reconstruction

Several methods for the reconstruction of gastrointestinal continuity have been described as follows [6, 7, 18–20]: gastroduodenostomy, gastrojejunostomy, or Roux-en-Y gastrojejunostomy; intracorporeal or extracorporeal; and linear or circular staplers including transoral anvil placement (Orvil). Because each reconstruction method has its advantages and shortcomings, the selection of the method depends on the resection extent and surgeon's preference based on their experience. In addition, when an endoscopic linear stapler that can be attached to the robotic arm will be available, robotic approach for intracorporeal anastomosis will be easier and more comfortable.

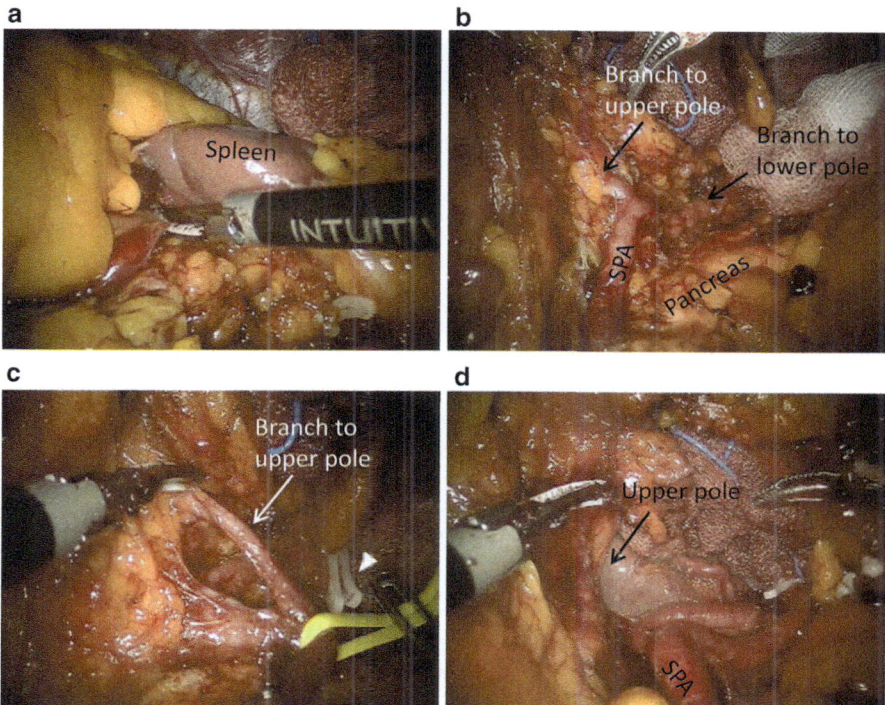

Fig. 5.8 Lymph node dissection of the splenic hilum during spleen-preserving total gastrectomy. (**a**) It is necessary to exchange the ultrasonic shears and Maryland bipolar forceps when the distance between the port of the 2nd arm and the splenic hilum is too long for ultrasonic shears to reach. (**b**) The proximal portion of the branches of splenic vessels at the splenic hilar area is exposed. (**c**). The branches of splenic vessels are exposed from lower to upper polar vessels. (**d**). Completed lymph node dissection of the splenic hilum during spleen-preserving total gastrectomy. *SPA* splenic artery

5.4 Review of Clinical Studies

Robotic approach for surgical treatment of gastric cancer offered ergonomic and technical benefits to surgeons. Using these advantages, surgeons have made efforts to overcome the shortcomings of conventional laparoscopic approach, especially in radical lymph node dissection that is required from the viewpoint of oncologic principles. Several studies comparing robotic gastrectomy to conventional laparoscopic gastrectomy have been reported, which showed acceptable short-term outcomes of robotic gastrectomy. However, because robotic gastrectomy is a relatively novel field for gastric cancer treatment, scientific evidence of the superiority of robotic approach to conventional laparoscopy is still lacking.

One of the largest comparative study published in 2011 [3] showed better short-term outcomes of robotic gastrectomy in terms of reduced intraoperative blood loss compared to conventional laparoscopy. This study also demonstrated its comparable oncologic outcomes to conventional laparoscopic gastrectomy, showing that the number of lymph nodes retrieved did not differ significantly between the two groups. Notably, no tumor involvement was observed in the resection line in the robotic group, while the laparoscopic group did not. The authors concluded that a robotic approach to gastric cancer is a promising alternative to conventional laparoscopic gastrectomy. A meta-analysis published in 2012 comparing robotic and laparoscopic gastrectomy for gastric cancer [21] revealed that robotic gastrectomy was significantly associated with less blood loss with an expense of longer operation time. It also showed comparable overall morbidity and mortality.

In a technical aspect, one single-center prospective case series demonstrated an integrated robotic approach of D2 lymphadenectomy for gastric cancer surgery, which showed no pancreas-related complications, although the number of patients was small [5]. Because pancreas-related complications were mostly associated with radical lymph node dissection, this study suggested the safety of peripancreatic lymphadenectomy using robotic approach.

Although no randomized controlled trial has been reported comparing robotic and laparoscopic gastrectomy, these reports support the feasibility of robotic gastrectomy for gastric cancer, provided that these operations are performed by experienced surgeons. Multicenter, randomized controlled trials are unequivocally required to establish the sound evidence of robotic gastrectomy in terms of both short- and long-term outcomes.

5.5 Advantages of Robotic Approach in Gastric Cancer Surgery

Considering radical lymph node dissection during gastrectomy, there are several difficulties in conventional laparoscopic gastrectomy [22, 23]. Especially in suprapancreatic lymph node dissection, it is technically challenging to keep the right plane of dissection between adipose tissues and major suprapancreatic vessels or pancreatic parenchyma because of surgeons' tremors and 2-D flat views. Furthermore, it is also difficult for surgeons to reach the deep portion of the suprapancreatic area with straight instruments without internal articulation for conventional laparoscopic surgery. Nevertheless, for oncologically complete D2 lymphadenectomy, it is necessary to retrieve lymphatic tissues located in the dorsal side of suprapancreatic vessels. Thus, some experienced surgeons started to employ robotic gastrectomy as a promising alternative to conventional laparoscopic gastrectomy [3–8].

The robotic surgery system is able to facilitate technically and oncologically safe robotic gastrectomy, especially in suprapancreatic lymph node dissection, by offering potential benefits to gastric surgeons, such as steady 3D images, an intuitive movement of robot arm instruments, tremor filtering, motion scaling, and instruments with articulating function with 7 degrees of freedom. Robotic articulated instruments make it easier for surgeons to reach the deep dorsal portion of suprapancreatic area compared to laparoscopic unarticulated instruments. Due to stable retraction of tissues by robotic instruments without tremor, surgeons can reduce potential risk of injury to lymphatic tissues and bleeding from dissection plane.

Robotic approach may also enable surgeons to carry out sufficient dissection of lymph node #10, which is located at the splenic hilum, during spleen-preserving total gastrectomy with D2 lymphadenectomy. Complicated vascular anatomy at the splenic hilum sometimes makes surgeons troubled in dissecting lymph node #10. The small branches of the splenic vessels may compromise sufficient lymphadenectomy in the area of the splenic hilum by frequently causing intraoperative hemorrhage. However, the mechanical advantages of robotic approach listed above allow surgeons to easily dissect along the splenic vessels and to sufficiently clear the lymphatic tissue with minimal intraoperative hemorrhage.

By using a robotic surgery system, gastric cancer surgeons can potentially overcome difficulties of D2 lymphadenectomy during MIS. However, robotic surgery has several disadvantages such as expensive initial cost of robot for hospitals, extra financial burden for patients, and longer operative time [3, 21]. It is still controversial whether these disadvantages of robotic approach can be justified by the advantages in radical lymphadenectomy. Future randomized controlled trials should be warranted to assess whether these robotic advantages are beneficial for long-term clinical outcomes of gastric cancer patients.

5.6 Conclusions

In this chapter, we demonstrated the procedures, current status, and clinical advantages of robotic gastrectomy for gastric cancer. Robotic gastrectomy with radical lymphadenectomy is considered as a safe and feasible alternative to conventional laparoscopy. Although scientific evidence of superiority to conventional laparoscopic surgery is still lacking, robotic gastrectomy for gastric cancer patients may be a promising approach by offering more accurate and delicate lymphadenectomy to the patients, which might improve short- and long-term outcomes of gastric cancer patients.

References

1. Kitano S, Iso Y, Moriyama M et al (1994) Laparoscopy-assisted Billroth I gastrectomy. Surg Laparosc Endosc 4:146–148
2. Kim HH, Hyung WJ, Cho GS et al (2010) Morbidity and mortality of laparoscopic gastrectomy versus open gastrectomy for gastric cancer: an interim report–a phase III multicenter, prospective, randomized trial (KLASS Trial). Ann Surg 251:417–420
3. Woo Y, Hyung WJ, Pak KH et al (2011) Robotic gastrectomies offer a sound oncologic surgical alternative for the treatment of early gastric cancers comparing favorably with laparoscopic resections. Arch Surg 146:1086–1092

4. D'Annibale A, Pende V, Pernazza G et al (2011) Full robotic gastrectomy with extended (D2) lymphadenectomy for gastric cancer: surgical technique and preliminary results. J Surg Res 166:e113–e120
5. Uyama I, Kanaya S, Ishida Y et al (2012) Novel integrated robotic approach for suprapancreatic D2 nodal dissection for treating gastric cancer: technique and initial experience. World J Surg 36:331–337
6. Kim MC, Heo GU, Jung GJ (2010) Robotic gastrectomy for gastric cancer: surgical techniques and clinical merits. Surg Endosc 24:610–615
7. Song J, Oh SJ, Kang WH et al (2009) Robot-assisted gastrectomy with lymph node dissection for gastric cancer: lessons learned from an initial 100 consecutive procedures. Ann Surg 249:927–932
8. Anderson C, Ellenhorn J, Hellan M et al (2007) Pilot series of robot-assisted laparoscopic subtotal gastrectomy with extended lymphadenectomy for gastric cancer. Surg Endosc 21:1662–1666
9. Kim KM, An JY, Kim HI et al (2012) Major early complications following open, laparoscopic and robotic gastrectomy. Br J Surg 99:1681–1687
10. Hashizume M, Sugimachi K (2003) Robot-assisted gastric surgery. Surg Clin N Am 83:1429–1444
11. Woo Y, Hyung WJ, Kim HI et al (2011) Minimizing hepatic trauma with a novel liver retraction method: a simple liver suspension using gauze suture. Surg Endosc 25:3939–3945
12. Shinohara T, Kanaya S, Yoshimura F et al (2011) A protective technique for retraction of the liver during laparoscopic gastrectomy for gastric adenocarcinoma: using a Penrose drain. J Gastrointest Surg 15:1043–1048
13. Kinjo Y, Okabe H, Obama K et al (2011) Elevation of liver function tests after laparoscopic gastrectomy using a Nathanson liver retractor. World J Surg 35:2730–2738
14. Hur H, Jeon HM, Kim W (2008) Laparoscopic pancreas- and spleen-preserving D2 lymph node dissection in advanced (cT2) upper-third gastric cancer. J Surg Oncol 97:169–172
15. Hyung WJ, Lim JS, Song J et al (2008) Laparoscopic spleen-preserving splenic hilar lymph node dissection during total gastrectomy for gastric cancer. J Am Coll Surg 207:e6–e11
16. Sakuramoto S, Kikuchi S, Futawatari N et al (2009) Laparoscopy-assisted pancreas- and spleen-preserving total gastrectomy for gastric cancer as compared with open total gastrectomy. Surg Endosc 23:2416–2423
17. Marano A, Hyung WJ (2012) Robotic gastrectomy: the current state of the art. J Gastric Cancer 12:63–72
18. Hyung WJ, Woo YH, Noh SH (2011) Robotic surgery for gastric cancer: a technical review. J Robot Surg 5:241–249
19. Pugliese R, Maggioni D, Sansonna F et al (2009) Outcomes and survival after laparoscopic gastrectomy for adenocarcinoma. Analysis on 65 patients operated on by conventional or robot-assisted minimal access procedures. Eur J Surg Oncol 35:281–288
20. Pugliese R, Maggioni D, Sansonna F et al (2010) Subtotal gastrectomy with D2 dissection by minimally invasive surgery for distal adenocarcinoma of the stomach: results and 5-year survival. Surg Endosc 24:2594–2602
21. Xiong B, Ma L, Zhang C et al (2012) Robotic versus laparoscopic gastrectomy for gastric cancer: a meta-analysis of short outcomes. Surg Oncol 21:274–280
22. Noshiro H, Nagai E, Shimizu S et al (2005) Laparoscopically assisted distal gastrectomy with standard radical lymph node dissection for gastric cancer. Surg Endosc 19:1592–1596
23. Song KY, Kim SN, Park CH (2008) Laparoscopy-assisted distal gastrectomy with D2 lymph node dissection for gastric cancer: technical and oncologic aspects. Surg Endosc 22:655–659

Esophageal Cancer Surgery

Robotic Esophagectomy in the Prone Position

Koichi Suda and Ichiro Uyama

Abbreviations

ICS	Intercostal space
R1	The 1st arm
R2	The 2nd arm
R3	The 3rd arm
RLN	Recurrent laryngeal nerve
RLNP	Recurrent laryngeal nerve palsy

6.1 Introduction

Esophageal cancer is the eighth most common cancer in the world. Asian countries including Japan have the highest incidence rates and the most common type of esophageal cancers in this region is squamous cell carcinoma [1]. Esophagectomy with total mediastinal lymphadenectomy with or without cervical lymphadenectomy, which has been recognized as radical esophagectomy, remains the main option for the curative treatment of esophageal squamous cell carcinoma [2, 3]. However, meticulous mediastinal lymph node dissection, especially along the left recurrent laryngeal nerve (RLN), frequently induces recurrent laryngeal nerve palsy (RLNP), leading to postoperative laryngopharyngeal dysfunction [4]. As a matter of fact, the incidence of RLNP following radical esophagectomy has been reported to range at a rate of up to 80 % [4].

K. Suda, M.D., Ph.D. • I. Uyama, M.D., Ph.D., FACS (✉)
Division of Upper GI, Department of Surgery, Fujita Health University, 1-98 Dengakugakubo, Kutsukake, Toyoake, Aichi 470-1192, Japan
e-mail: iuyama@fujita-hu.ac.jp

Thoracoscopic radical esophagectomy in the prone position with carbon dioxide insufflation has been demonstrated to provide excellent surgical field around the left RLN with sufficient short-term outcomes [5]. Surgical robots have been developed to overcome some of the disadvantages of standard minimally invasive surgery such as two-dimensional image with poor depth perception, long-handled forceps with the limited degree of freedom, shaking of the surgeon's hand, and limited tactile sensation [6]. As a result, surgical robots facilitate precise dissection in a confined surgical field with impressive dexterity [4, 6]. Thus, in 2009, we started using the robotic system in thoracoscopic esophagectomy in the prone position and have demonstrated the possibility that the use of the robotic system in thoracoscopic esophagectomy in the prone position might reduce postoperative laryngopharyngeal dysfunction related to RLNP [4]. In this chapter, we present our latest methods and short-term outcomes of robotic esophagectomy.

6.2 Methods

6.2.1 Patients

All the operative patients with resectable esophageal squamous cell carcinoma who had not undergone prior gastrectomy were evenly offered robotic surgery. Patients who agreed to uninsured use of da Vinci S HD Surgical System underwent robotic esophagectomy with total mediastinal lymphadenectomy in the prone position. The stage of the cancer was described according to the Japanese Classification of Esophageal Cancer, the 10th edition, revised version [7].

6.2.2 Patient's Position

The patient was initially placed in the prone position under a combination of general and intravenous anesthesia and using a double-lumen endotracheal tube for single-lung ventilation. The right arm was raised cranially to expose the right axillar fossa. The face was placed toward the right to facilitate suction of the sputa by bronchial scope and to avoid increasing ophthalmic pressure (Fig. 6.1). All surgeons stood on the right chest side of the patient, and a high-quality video monitor was set up on the opposite side (Fig. 6.2).

6.2.3 Trocar Arrangement

The distance between the operated target and the camera trocar has to be longer than one hand, and that between each trocar has to be longer than 4 digits. We have currently been using the 6-port system. In particular, we fully utilized the 3rd arm (R3) by docking it to the trocar placed in the 3rd intercostal space (ICS), because we believed that R3 is especially useful for upper mediastinal lymph node dissection.

6 Esophageal Cancer Surgery

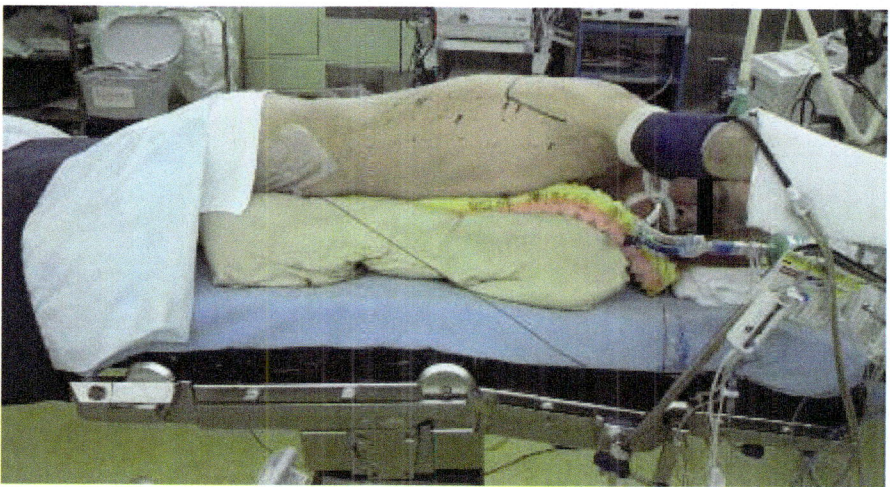

Fig. 6.1 Patient's position for robotic esophagectomy

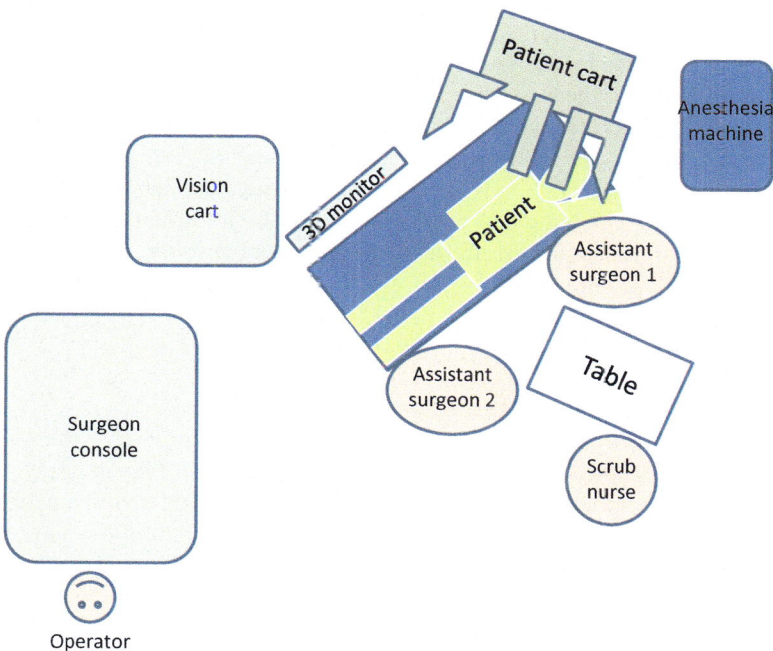

Fig. 6.2 The setup and positioning of the operating team in the use of the robotic esophagectomy in the prone position

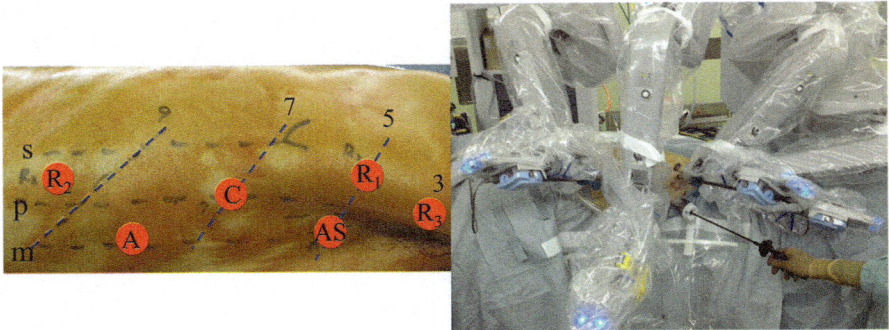

Fig. 6.3 Trocar arrangement for robotic esophagectomy in the prone position. *s* scapula angle line, *p* posterior axillary line, *m* midaxillary line, *3* 3rd ICS, *5* 5th ICS, *7* 7th ICS, *9* 9th ICS, R_1 1st arm, R_2 2nd arm, R_3 3rd arm, *A* assistant surgeon, *C* camera, *AS* AirSeal, *ICS* intercostal space

In detail, a 12-mm blunt trocar for the thoracoscope was inserted into the 7th ICS on the posterior axillary line, carefully confirming the absence of pleural adhesion. Another five trocars were inserted under thoracoscopic guidance: an 8-mm trocar in the 3rd ICS on the posterior axillary line for R3, an 8-mm trocar in the 5th ICS on the scapula angle line for the 1st arm (R1), a 12-mm trocar in the 8th ICS behind the midaxillary line for the assistant, an 8-mm trocar in the 10th ICS behind the posterior axillary line for the 2nd arm (R2), and a 14-mm AirSeal Access Port in the 5th ICS behind the midaxillary line for AirSeal System (SurgiQuest Inc., Milford, Connecticut, USA) to achieve stable carbon dioxide insufflation with decreased camera smudging and better vision (Fig. 6.3). Carbon dioxide pneumothorax was achieved at a pressure of 6 mmHg to collapse the right lung and to expand the mediastinum.

6.2.4 Docking of the Patient Cart

Regarding the docking of the patient cart, the sagittal plane of its mainstay, which we termed as "da Vinci's axis," is very important. To prevent a collision between R1 and R3 during lymph node dissection along the right recurrent laryngeal nerve, the patient cart had to dock with the patient over the patient's left shoulder with da Vinci's axis on the line connecting between the right subclavicular artery and the camera trocar (Fig. 6.4). When this setup induced a collision between R1 and the camera during lower mediastinal lymph node dissection, the patient cart was undocked and redocked with da Vinci's axis on the line connecting between the arch of the azygos vein and the camera trocar.

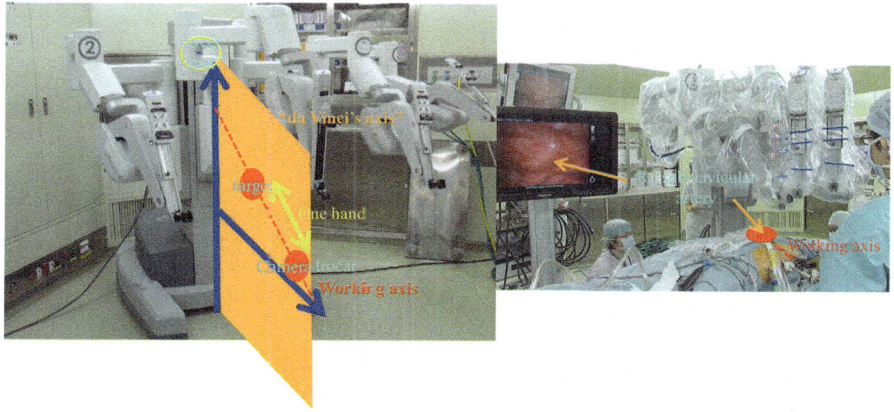

Fig. 6.4 Optimal manner of docking of the patient cart using "da Vinci's axis" in the use of robotic esophagectomy in the prone position

6.2.5 Forceps and Energy Devices

The operator used Maryland bipolar forceps (420172, Intuitive) or monopolar curved scissors (420179, Intuitive) for cutting and coagulation with R1 or R3, fenestrated bipolar forceps (420205, Intuitive) for hemostasis with R2, and Cadiere forceps (420049, Intuitive) with R3 or R1. VIO® 300 D Electrosurgical Unit (ERBE, Marietta, Georgia, USA) was used as an electrosurgical generator.

6.2.6 Thoracoscopic Surgical Procedures in the Prone Position

We usually dissect the right bronchial artery and preserve the left bronchial artery and the thoracic duct.

6.2.6.1 Mobilization of the Anterior Aspect of the Middle and Lower Thoracic Esophagus on the Dorsal Aspect of the Pericardium

The right lower pulmonary ligament was dissected and the mediastinal pleura overlying the anterior aspect of the lower and middle thoracic esophagus was opened. The anterior aspect of the lower and middle thoracic esophagus was widely mobilized on the dorsal aspect of the pericardium. The anterior aspect of the right main bronchus nodes (#109R) and the middle thoracic esophagus was mobilized from the pericardium. The right pulmonary vein was exposed (Fig. 6.5). Then, #109R was dissected along the right main bronchus. The distal side of the right bronchial artery was divided and transected, preserving the pulmonary branch of the right vagus nerve. The bifurcation nodes (#107) were subsequently dissected.

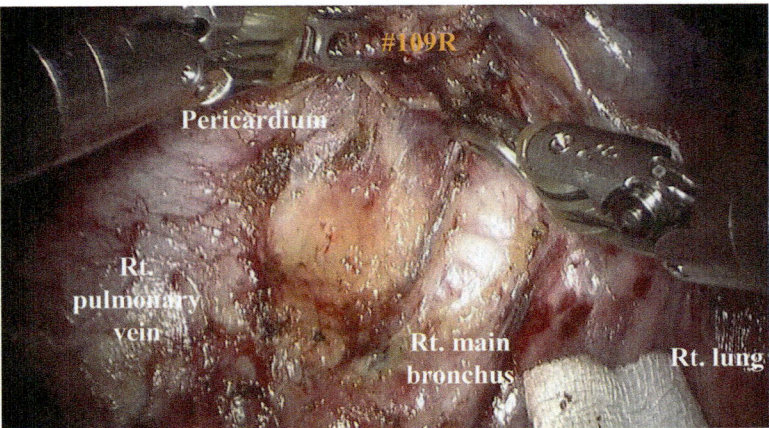

Fig. 6.5 Mobilization of the anterior aspect of the middle and lower thoracic esophagus on the dorsal aspect of the pericardium, #109R and 107 lymph node dissection

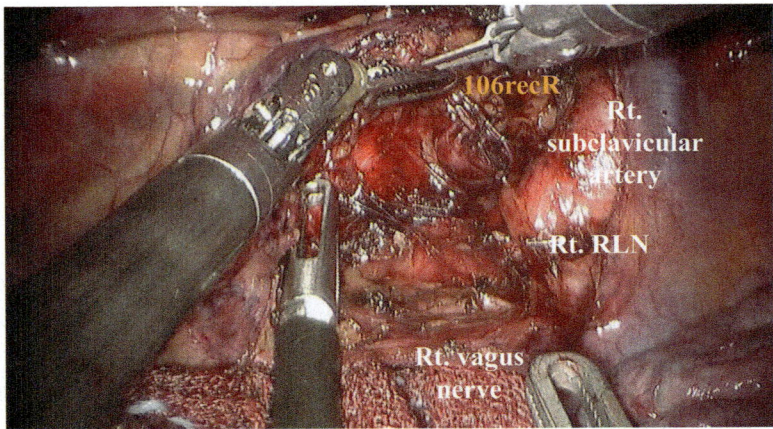

Fig. 6.6 Lymph node dissection along the right recurrent laryngeal nerve, RLN

6.2.6.2 Right Upper Mediastinal Procedures: #106recR+101 R Dissection

The pleura overlying the anterior aspect of the upper thoracic esophagus was opened along the right vagus nerve. Upper thoracic paraesophageal nodes (#105) were dissected along the right vagus nerve. Then, the right RLN was exposed on the right subclavicular artery. The lymph nodes around the right RLN (#106recR +101R) were sharply dissected near below the thyroid gland through the thoracic inlet without using electrocautery to avoid injury (Fig. 6.6). Esophageal branches of the right RLN were divided in turn.

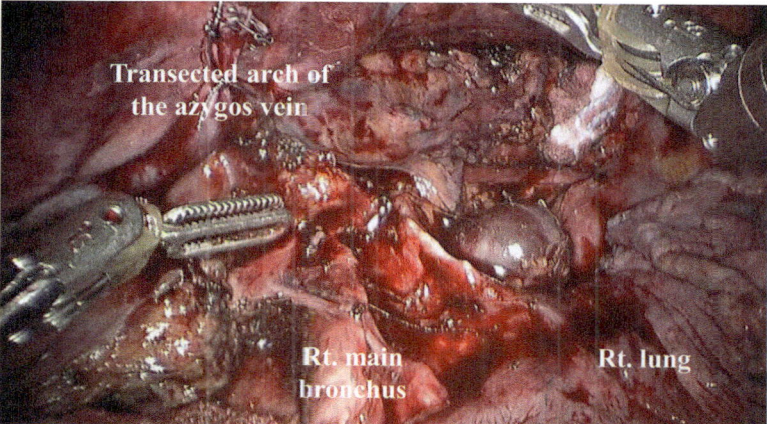

Fig. 6.7 Operative field after transection of the arch of the azygos vein

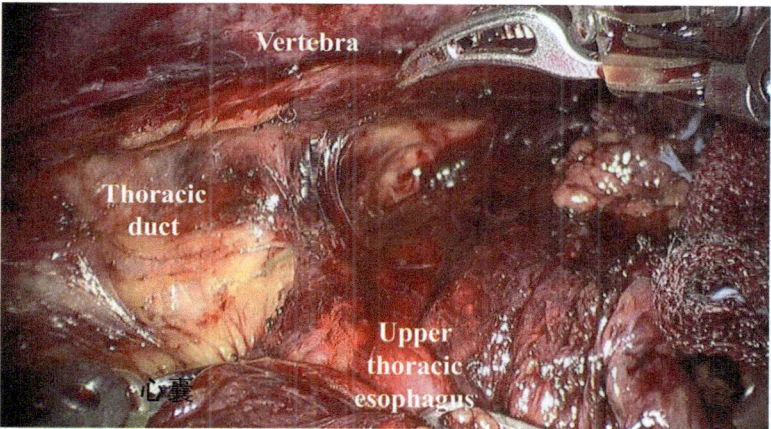

Fig. 6.8 Mobilization of the posterior aspect of the upper thoracic esophagus carefully preserving the thoracic duct

6.2.6.3 Transection of the Arch of the Azygos Vein

The pleura overlying the posterior aspect of the upper thoracic esophagus was opened. Then, the pleura covering the arch of the azygos vein was cut. The arch of the azygos vein was transected with a linear stapler and the distal edge was pulled to the back with a stitch (Fig. 6.7).

6.2.6.4 Mobilization of the Posterior Aspect of the Upper and Middle Thoracic Esophagus on a Vascular Sheath Covering the Aortic Arch and the Left Subclavicular Artery

The posterior aspect of the upper and middle thoracic esophagus was mobilized on a vascular sheath of the dense connective tissue covering the aortic arch and the left subclavicular artery, carefully preserving the thoracic duct (Fig. 6.8). The left

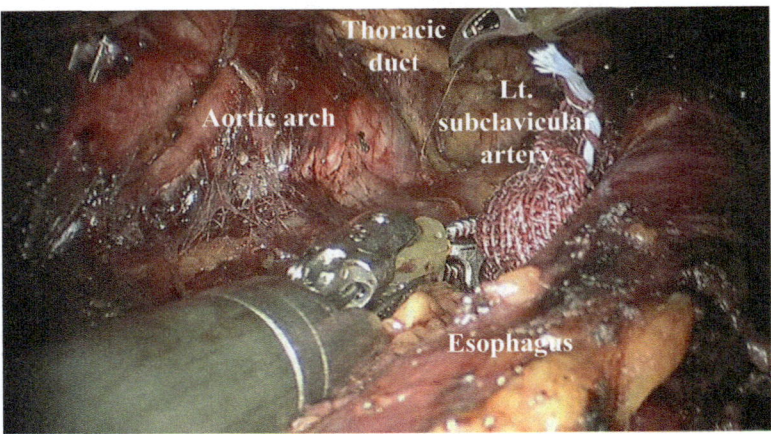

Fig. 6.9 Mobilization of the posterior aspect of the upper and middle thoracic esophagus on a vascular sheath covering the aortic arch and the left subclavicular artery

subclavicular artery was exposed (Fig. 6.9). Pleura overlying the posterior aspect of the middle thoracic esophagus was additionally opened and mobilization of the posterior aspect of the esophagus was continued. The origin of the right bronchial artery was divided. The descending aorta and the aortic arch were exposed.

6.2.6.5 Mobilization of the Anterior Aspect of the Middle and Upper Thoracic Esophagus and #105+108 Dissection

The anterior aspect of the left main bronchus nodes (#109 L) and the middle thoracic esophagus were mobilized on the pericardium. The left pulmonary vein was exposed. Then, upper and middle thoracic paraesophageal nodes (#105+108) were dissected along the right vagus nerve. Membranous portion of the trachea was exposed. Esophageal branches of the right vagus nerve were divided while preserving the pulmonary branches (Fig. 6.10).

6.2.6.6 Lymph Node Dissection Along the Left Recurrent Laryngeal Nerve (#106recL+101 L)

The main cuff of a double-lumen endotracheal tube was deflated temporarily and the trachea was rolled back carefully and firmly to the right and ventrally by a grasper holding small gauze to explore the left aspect of the trachea and the left main bronchus. The anterior aspect of the upper thoracic esophagus was released from the membranous portion of the trachea toward the neck to allow for a sufficient number of lymph nodes up to the thoracic inlet to be dissected. Adipose tissue including #106recR+101R and #105 was detached out of the upper thoracic esophagus. Then, the adipose tissue including the left RLN and the left paratracheal nodes (#106recL) was dissected along the left aspect of the trachea and the left bronchus. The left cervical paraesophageal nodes (#101 L) were additionally dissected. Some esophageal or tracheal branches of the identified left RLN were

6 Esophageal Cancer Surgery

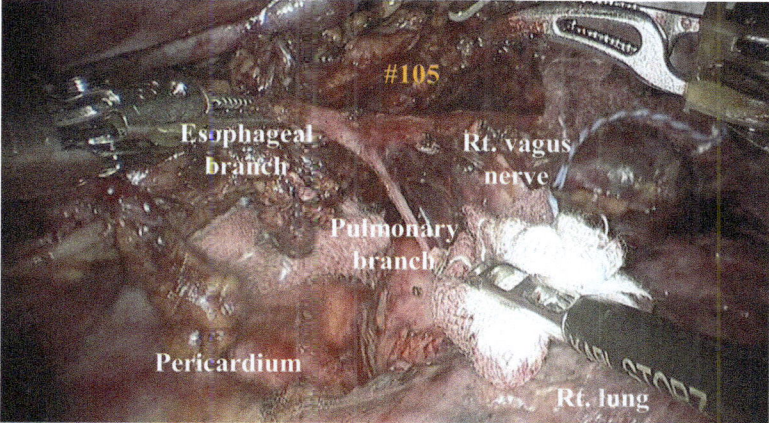

Fig. 6.10 Esophageal branches of the right vagus nerve

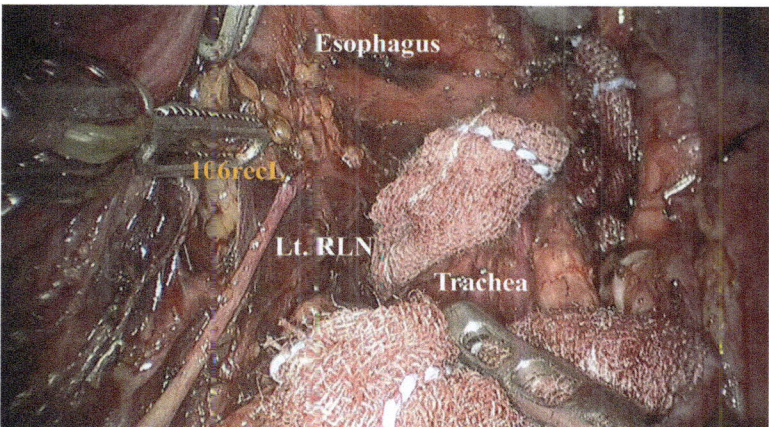

Fig. 6.11 Lymph node dissection along the left recurrent laryngeal nerve, RLN

divided. The left RLN was sharply isolated from the explored tissue without using electrocautery to avoid injury, and finally, the anterior aspect of #106recL+101 L was dissected (Fig. 6.11).

6.2.6.7 Dissection of the Infra-Aortic Arch Nodes

Adipose tissue including #106recL+101 L and #105 was detached out of the upper thoracic esophagus. The upper thoracic esophagus was mobilized circumferentially, and the esophagus was divided at the level of the aortic arch by linear stapling. The infra-aortic arch nodes (#106tbL) were dissected on the face of the pulmonary artery trunk, preserving the recurrent portion of the left recurrent laryngeal nerve, left vagus nerve, and one or two left bronchial arteries (Fig. 6.12).

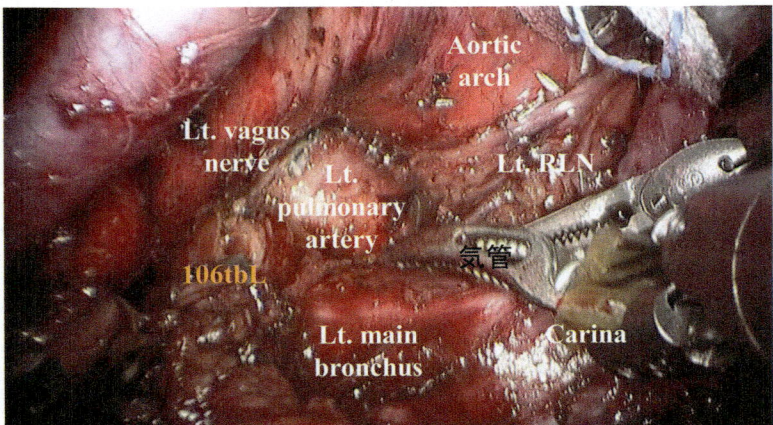

Fig. 6.12 Dissection of the infra-aortic arch nodes (#106 tbL) on the face of the pulmonary artery trunk

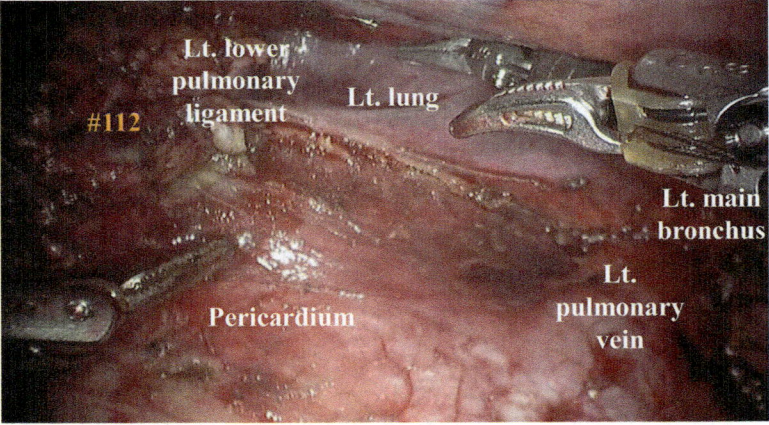

Fig. 6.13 Dissection of the lower posterior mediastinal nodes

6.2.6.8 Dissection of the Lower Posterior Mediastinal Nodes

The caudal side of the divided esophagus was dissected on the membranous portion of the left bronchus. The esophageal branches of the left vagus nerve were dissected. #109 L was removed from the left main bronchus. Carefully preserving the thoracic duct, lower posterior mediastinal nodes (#112) were dissected on the pericardium, descending aorta, left pleura, and diaphragm. Left pleura was opened and the left inferior pulmonary ligament was dissected (Fig. 6.13). Diaphragmatic crus was exposed circumferentially and #111 was dissected.

6.2.6.9 Completion of the Thoracic Phase

After the thoracoscopic procedures were completed, a 19Fr Blake drain (Ethicon, Somerville, NJ, USA) was inserted. The reconstruction of an alimentary tract was done at the neck between the cervical esophagus and a gastric conduit which was created with laparoscopic assistance. To do this, a long plastic bag through which a cotton tape passes was placed in the posterior mediastinum when thoracic phase was completed. The cranial end of the bag was sutured to the cranial end of the divided esophagus and pulled out of the cervical wound, and the other end was sutured to the caudal end of the divided esophagus and pulled out of the abdominal wound. Then, the caudal end of the cotton tape was sutured to the gastric conduit and the other end was reeled to pull up the gastric conduit through the posterior mediastinum [4]. In this series, cervical paraesophageal nodes (#101) were dissected through the thoracic inlet in the thoracic phase, and internal jugular and supraclavicular nodes (#102+104) were not dissected.

6.3 Results

Twenty-three patients have undergone robotic esophagectomy with reconstruction using a gastric conduit at Fujita Health University Hospital, so far. Patient background factors were as follows: male/female, 21:2; age 65 (50–86); tumor size 3.5 (0.9–10) cm; tumor location Ut: Mt: Lt, 3:11:9; and pathological stage 0: I: II: III: IVa, 6:3:4:7:3. Seven patients underwent preoperative chemotherapy or chemoradiation therapy. Surgical outcomes were as follows: operation time, thoracic phase 367 (206–492) m, total 710 (536–834) m; blood loss, thoracic phase 79 (0–206) mL, total 193 (20–502) mL; the number of dissected lymph nodes, thoracic 21 (11–39), total 41 (23–63); and completeness of resection, R0: R1, 21:2. Sixteen patients developed postoperative complications including vocal cord palsy in ten patients, aspiration in nine patients, hoarseness in seven patients, anastomotic leakage in six patients, pneumonia in three patients, and arrhythmia in two patients. Duration of ventilator dependency was 0.5 (0–2.5) day, ICU stay was 0.5 (0–8.5) day, and hospital stay following surgery was 24 (7–67) days. There was no in-hospital mortality in this series.

6.4 Discussion

Our previous study demonstrated that the use of the surgical robot in esophagectomy might reduce recurrent laryngeal nerve palsy and help preserve laryngopharyngeal function, leading to the improvement in the short-term postoperative course, compared to the standard minimally invasive approach [4]. There were no significant differences in operation time, blood loss, the number of dissected lymph nodes, completeness of resection, and the other complications unrelated to laryngeal nerve palsy [4]. Robot assistance might be a promising minimally invasive approach to perform thoracoscopic total mediastinal lymphadenectomy, even though there have been a couple of issues to be solved such as long operation time, high cost, and unclear long-term outcomes [4, 6].

Acknowledgments This work was not supported by any grants and fundings. No author has commercial association with or financial involvement that might pose a conflict of interest in connection with the submitted article.

References

1. Eslick GD (2009) Epidemiology of esophageal cancer. Gastroenterol Clin North Am 38:17–25
2. Fujita H, Sueyoshi S, Tanaka T et al (2002) Three-field dissection for squamous cell carcinoma in the thoracic esophagus. Ann Thorac Cardiovasc Surg 8:328–335
3. Fumagalli U (1996) Panel of experts. Resective surgery for cancer of the thoracic esophagus: results of a consensus conference held at the 6th world congress of the international society for diseases of the Esophagus. Dis Esophagus 9(suppl):30–38
4. Suda K, Ishida Y, Kawamura Y, Inaba K, Kanaya S, Teramukai S, Satoh S, Uyama I (2012) Robot-assisted thoracoscopic lymphadenectomy along the left recurrent laryngeal nerve for esophageal squamous cell carcinoma in the prone position: technical report and short-term outcomes. World J Surg 36:1608–1616
5. Noshiro H, Iwasaki H, Kobayashi K et al (2010) Lymphadenectomy along the left recurrent laryngeal nerve by a minimally invasive esophagectomy in the prone position for thoracic esophageal cancer. Surg Endosc 24:2965–2973
6. Uyama I, Suda K, Satoh S (2013) Laparoscopic surgery for advanced gastric cancer: current status and future perspectives. J Gastric Cancer, 13:19–25
7. Japanese Esophageal Society (2008) Japanese classification of esophageal cancer, the 10th edn. revised version, Kanehara Shuppan, Tokyo

7. Lateral Pelvic Node Dissection for Advanced Rectal Cancer: Current Debates and Use of the Robotic Approach

Gyu-Seog Choi

7.1 Introduction

While lateral lymphatic drainage of the rectum was identified as early as the 1920s [1–4], its importance in the treatment of rectal cancer has been primarily studied by Japanese surgeons [5–7]. Conversely, in the West, the value of neoadjuvant or adjuvant chemoradiation has been investigated by several clinical trials and proven to be an effective method of reducing the rate of local recurrence [8–10]. As a result, neoadjuvant chemoradiation with total mesorectal excision (TME) is considered standard treatment for advanced rectal cancer. Still, despite gradual adoption of radiation in Japan, lateral pelvic node dissection (LPND) is routinely recommended when the lower border of rectal cancer is located below the peritoneal reflection and the tumor has invaded beyond the proper muscle of the rectum [11].

Although many studies have been published reporting favorable results [12, 13] with minimally invasive surgery for rectal cancer, its oncologic safety remains to be proven via randomized clinical trials [14, 15]. Laparoscopic TME is in itself technically difficult, as is LPND, and for laparoscopic LPND, only a few sporadic reports give us any indication of its feasibility [16–18].

In recent years, robotic surgery using the da Vinci Surgical System has emerged as the next generation of minimally invasive surgery. With its use come many mechanical advantages over laparoscopy, including endo-wrist function of instruments to

G.-S. Choi, M.D., Ph.D. (✉)
Colorectal Cancer Center, Kyungpook National University Medical Center, School of Medicine, Kyungpook National University, 807 Hogukro, Buk-gu, Daegu 702-210, South Korea
e-mail: kyuschoi@mail.knu.ac.kr

improve degree of freedom in movement, fine movement without hand tremor to facilitate precise dissection, surgeon control of most of the instruments, a three-dimensional magnified surgical view, and more. Unfortunately, the da Vinci robotic system also comes with disadvantages, including limited range of surgical field, an intuitive but not versatile approach, and high costs.

Still, taken together with the pros and cons of the robotic system, rectal cancer could be one of the best indications for this new approach and even more suitable for LPND if we take into consideration the technical complexity and narrow anatomical space with important nerves and vessels. To date there has been little publication to evaluate feasibility and efficacy of robotic LPND, with the exception of our previous preliminary report [19].

Herein, the author reviews current debates regarding LPND, the surgical technique of robotic LPND, and its clinical results.

7.2 Anatomy of Lateral Pelvic Node

Lymphatic drainage of the rectum and anus was studied and described as early as the 1900s. Miles [1] first used the terms "upward," "downward," and "lateral" zone of lymphatic spread which, today, are equivalent to "superior rectal-inferior mesenteric" route, "ischiorectal-inguinal" route, and "internal, external iliac, obturator" route. In 1940, Coller [2] described a high incidence of lymph node metastasis from lower rectal cancer and emphasized the need to remove the lateral zone as well as the superior zone of lymph node in patients with lower rectal or anal cancer. On the opposite side of the world, Japanese doctor Senba [3] reported lymphatic flow of the rectum similar to those of the West via dissection work of fetal cadavers. Following Senba's work, Kuru [4] published an article on the importance of LPND and high ligation of the inferior mesenteric artery in order to treat advanced rectal cancer.

Although the use of LPND in the treatment of rectal cancer was initiated on both sides of the world, Japanese surgeons are regarded as having pioneered this technique. According to their description of the "zone of lateral pelvic node," it is composed of six zones: internal iliac, middle rectal, obturator, common iliac, external iliac, and the aortic bifurcation area [20, 21]. Additionally, the most common areas of metastasis in patients with lower rectal cancer are consistently reported in the literature as middle rectal, internal iliac, and obturator group [20, 21].

7.3 Incidence of Lateral Pelvic Node Metastasis in Rectal Cancer

The incidence of LPN metastasis varies according to individual studies. This is due primarily to the heterogeneity of the tumor location and different indications of LPND depending on the surgeon and/or institution. Most recently, early postoperative results from a Japanese clinical trial (JCOG0212) showed that the rate of LPN metastasis in stage II–III lower rectal cancer, without clinical enlargement of LPN, was 7.4 % [22]. In general, the higher incidence is anticipated by the advanced tumor and nodal stage, the lower tumor location, and, often, the female gender. In reviewing several reports, the overall rate of LPN positivity in lower rectal cancer ranges is approximately 10–25 % [7, 23–26].

The accuracy of clinical diagnosis for LPN involvement by preoperative radiologic studies is also not well defined. Akasu et al. [27] used high-resolution MRI to identify positive LPN, thereby reporting an 87 % overall accuracy rate and 14 % positive rate among 104 rectal cancer patients. This was in concordance with their 17 % of pathologic positivity from a previous report. Yano et al. [28] reported an exceptionally high rate of accuracy (95 % sensitivity and 94 % specificity) by using a conventional CT scan. Conversely, Arii et al. [29] demonstrated an overall accuracy of CT scan and MRI for LPN metastasis to be only 51 % and 64 %, respectively, thus indicating that preoperative radiologic modality may not be reliable enough, particularly following neoadjuvant radiation [30].

7.4 Involvement of the Lateral Pelvic Node: Regional or Systemic?

The AJCC 7th edition of TNM staging system [31] clearly indicated that internal iliac nodes are regional lymph nodes, despite the fact that dissection of this area is rarely conducted by surgeons outside of Japan. In fact, many doctors in the West still consider them to be beyond the regional lymphatic chain. In a Japanese nationwide multi-institutional study, Akiyoshi et al. [21] evaluated whether or not LPN metastasis was a systemic disease. They categorized internal iliac nodes as regional lymph nodes and the remaining area of LPN as external lateral pelvic nodes (Ext-LPN). They then found that the overall and cancer-specific survival rates of patients with metastasis of internal iliac nodes were similar to those in the N2a category by TNM stage and that those with Ext-LPN positive were similar to the N2b group. Consequently, they concluded that lymph nodes in both of these groups appeared to be regional and not systemic.

A study from Korea also suggested that clinically proven LPN metastasis is highly correlated with locoregional recurrence, without distant spread, and could, therefore, be a potentially curative regional disease rather than a sign of systemic disease [32]. Still, other reports have shown that the survival rate of patients who are LPN positive, even after complete LPND, is significantly shorter than those with mesorectal node metastasis. This also advocates for metastasis of LPN to be considered a systemic disease [33], though it is still a question that remains to be answered.

7.5 Role of LPND Versus Neoadjuvant Chemoradiation

While the impact of LPND for advanced lower rectal cancer has been controversial and debated among surgeons in the west and Japan, both sides agree that LPN metastasis in advanced lower rectal cancer is a realistic event and that removal of these positive nodes may be beneficial for the patient. In western countries, however, surgeons believe that rectal cancer with metastasis of LPN is no longer considered a localized disease but rather a systemic one. They also view neoadjuvant chemoradiation as effective as LPND and believe that LPND is a demanding procedure that creates a longer operative time, excessive hemorrhaging, and a higher rate of severe morbidities, including genitourinary dysfunction due to injury of autonomic pelvic splanchnic nerves [34–36].

There have been several large-scale randomized clinical trials to support the promising role of chemoradiotherapy (CCRT) in controlling locoregional relapse following rectal cancer surgery [8–10]. Kuster et al. [37] reported a case-matched comparative study of Japanese TME + LPND without radiation versus Dutch TME + preoperative RT versus Dutch TME-only group. They found that the 5-year local recurrence rate of Japanese TME + LPND and Dutch TME + RT were not that different, at 6.9 % and 5.8 %, respectively. In fact, for lateral pelvic recurrence following either of these treatments, the rate was not significantly different between the groups. Additionally, although the Japanese group showed a significantly higher overall survival rate, they believe the preoperative CCRT could play a role as effectively as LPND did, with regard to local control of the rectal cancer. Kim et al. [38] also compared their results of TME + postoperative radiation in advanced lower rectal cancer with those of the Japanese TME + LPND group. They concluded that the local recurrence rate in stage III after Japanese TME + LPND was 2.2 times higher than that of TME + postoperative RT. Thus, even after LPND, adjuvant treatment such as radiation therapy could be recommended. Similarly, Watanabe et al. [24] found in their retrospective study to compare data from RT ± LPND and non-RT ± LPND groups (2 × 2 subgroup analysis) that the local recurrence after RT-LPND was the same as with non-RT + LPND. Finally, a meta-analysis [36] suggested that LPND showed no significant benefit in survival or disease-free survival, but did result in longer operative times, more blood loss, and a higher rate of morbidity, in particular, urinary dysfunction.

On the other hand, there have been a number of reports advocating the effectiveness of LPND, primarily from Japanese surgeons. In 2006, Sugihara's Japanese multicenter retrospective study reported that positive LPN was an independent prognostic factor and that LPND could reduce local recurrence in T3/T4 lower rectal cancer by 50.3 %, and improve 5-year survival rates by 8 % [39]. This data became part of the evidence used in the Japanese Society for Cancer of the Colon and Rectum (JSCCR) guidelines in 2010, for the treatment of colorectal cancer [11]. Fujita et al. [23] also noted the value of LPND in selective stage III cases with a small number of metastatic lymph nodes. He found the 5-year disease-free survival of patients with LPND was better than that found in the non-LPND group.

More recently, Kim et al. [32] described the importance of LPN metastasis, even after preoperative CRT. They found that lateral pelvic recurrence was a major pattern of local relapse following preoperative CRT + TME in advanced lower rectal cancer. More interestingly, 41.6 % of lateral pelvic recurrence showed no distant metastasis which speaks to the necessity of LPND, particularly in patients with clinically suspected LPNs larger than 5–10 mm in diameter, as found by preoperative imaging studies.

It can be concluded then that without prospective a randomized controlled study comparing the results of CRT and LPND, preoperative CRT cannot be viewed as able to eradicate metastatic LPN. Likewise, routine LPND alone appears to be an over-treatment due to the low rate of positive LPN. It seems reasonable then that selective LPND, in patients with unresolved swelling of LPN following preoperative CRT, can be viewed as an alternative solution to the two extremes.

7.6   Laparoscopic LPND

Today, the use of laparoscopic surgery for colorectal cancer continues to increase, though there are limited numbers of reports to be reviewed on the topic. Among them, the largest series was reported by Liang [17] who performed laparoscopic LPND in 34 selected patients of rectal cancer with sustained enlargement of LPN, even after preoperative CRT. The median operative time and blood loss for each LPND was 58 min and 44 mL, respectively. The incidence of positive lymph nodes among 45 LPNDs in 34 patients was very high at 71.1 %. During the 24-month follow-up period, there were nine (27.3 %) recurrences, including two local recurrences. During this same time, we reported our first laparoscopic LPND experience in 16 patients, including 2 robotic cases [18]. The indications were similar to Liang's with regard to selection criteria for LPND. The total operative time and blood loss was 310 min and 188 mL, respectively. Metastasis was identified in 56 % of patients who underwent LPND. During the follow-up period (median 32 months), 25 % of patients presented with distal recurrences and 12.5 % with local recurrences. Konish et al. [16] briefly described their results of laparoscopic LPND following preoperative CRT. In their study, the operative time and blood loss were 413 min and 25 mL, respectively. In 57.1 % of patients, metastasis of LPN was found. During a short follow-up period of 17 months, there were no recurrences or mortalities.

Laparoscopic LPND has been performed only in a few institutions and no comparative studies are available to date. As a result, it is too early to draw any conclusions beyond its technical feasibility.

7.7 Robotic LPND

7.7.1 Techniques of Robotic LPND

The technique of robotic LPND is similar to the laparoscopic approach, as we have previously described [19]. The patient is placed in a modified lithotomy position with both arms at the patient's side. We use a hybrid method which facilitates the laparoscopic splenic flexure take down and is followed by robotic rectal resection and LPND. Recently, we changed the port setup to add a single-incision multi-port (OCTO port®, South Korea) at the right lower quadrant of the abdominal wall, through which we effectively use the robotic instruments, assistant's graspers, and suction irrigator, as well as the linear stapler for rectal division. We also use that as a port for specimen retrieval and a protective ileostomy when indicated (Figs. 7.1 and 7.2). The robot is placed and engaged between the legs of the patient but slightly angled along the left thigh for access to the perineal area during the surgery.

The dissection of lateral nodes commences after the completion of TME and transection of the distal rectum. The first robot arm (with monopolar curved scissors) is used to perform the dissection. The second arm (with bipolar Cadiere forceps) is used to grasp and retract the lymphoareolar tissue and is sometimes used as an energy device in order to control bleeding. The third arm (with double-fenestrated grasper) has the most important function in this procedure, as it facilitates major traction to obtain surgical view. Additional retraction and fluid removal from the surgical field are provided by the assistant surgeon.

The actual LPND is started to isolate the ureter, hypogastric nerve, and pelvic nerves from the pelvic side wall. Thereafter, the dissection of lymph nodes is initiated at the area around the common iliac artery, followed by dissection between the bifurcation, and then between the internal iliac vessels and the hypogastric nerve (Fig. 7.2a). While the parietal pelvic peritoneum is elevated over the area and pushed to the lateral side by the third robot arm, the monopolar scissors open the peritoneum and dissect the lymphoareolar tissue from the common iliac vessels. The dissection is then extended downward and laterally to unroof the obturator fossa enclosed by internal and external iliac vessels laterally and the pelvic bone and muscles at its bottom. Special care must be taken to not injure the obturator nerve and to preserve the superior vesical artery, unless it is invaded by metastatic nodes. The double-fenestrated grasper with jaws opened can effectively help the surgeon create a good surgical field by pushing the external iliac vessels, ureter, and branches of the internal iliac artery simultaneously (Fig. 7.2b). En bloc resection of the lymphoareolar tissue in each compartment is recommended, as opposed to picking nodes up individually (Fig. 7.2c). The most common site of metastasis, around the middle rectal artery, can be reached by continuing dissection further down until the narrow space between the terminal branches of the internal iliac vessels and the bony pelvis are secured, along with the space between those vessels and pelvic nerves (Fig. 7.2b, c, d).

In cases with massive lymph nodes along the internal iliac vessels, removal of the contiguous two compartments of internal iliac and obturator group, and

Fig. 7.1 (a) Port setup. RC, robotic camera; R1, robotic arm 1; R2, robotic arm 2; R3, robotic arm 3; A1, assistant's port 1; A2, assistant's port 2. (b) External view of port setup

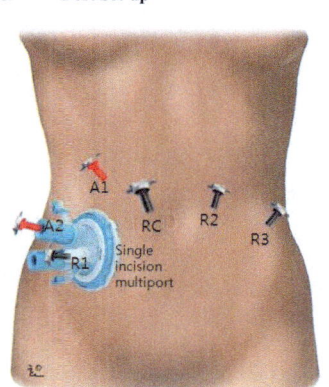

a   Port Set-up

RC: robotic camera,   R1: robotic arm 1, R2: robotic arm 2, R3: robotic arm 3

A1: assistant's port 1, A2: assistant's port 2

b   External view of port set-up

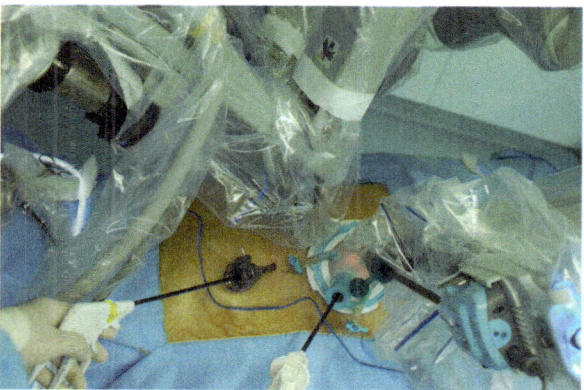

sacrificing their branches distal to the superior vesical artery, is recommended. In general, lymphadenectomy outside of the external iliac vessels and in the para-aortic area is not performed, with the exception of cases with highly suspicious metastatic nodes along those vessels.

In order to perform LPND effectively and safely, it is important to create a good surgical field using harmonious traction and counter-traction with a double-fenestrated grasper through the 3rd arm, the assistant's grasper through the right upper quadrant laparoscopic port, and a suction irrigator through one of the multi-port in single-incision access port used, on the right lower quadrant of the abdomen. It is also important to understand the design of the endo-wrist instruments and to know that the well-insulated energy source is one of the best technical tips for use in robotic LPND for precision and minimal bleeding.

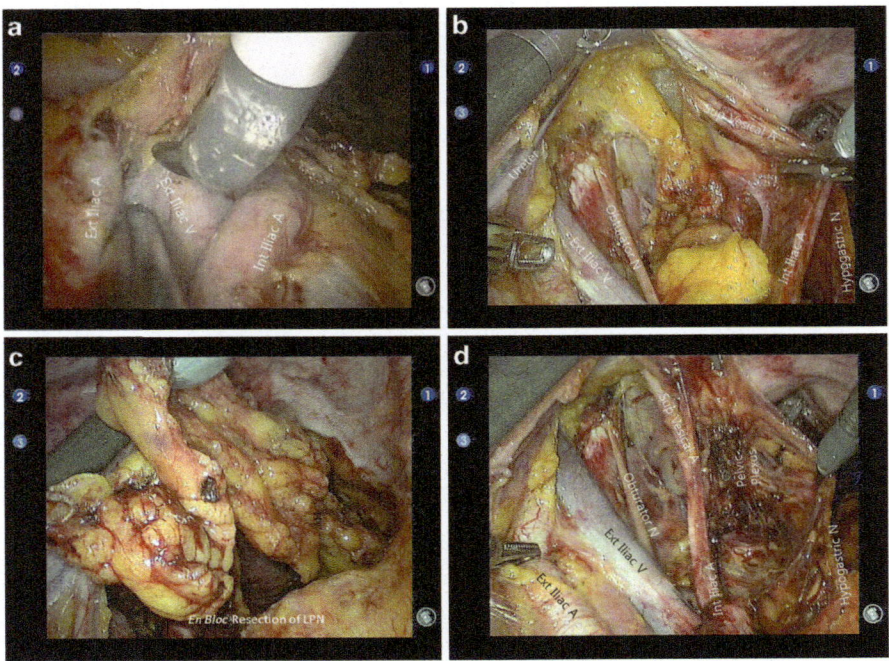

Fig. 7.2 Robotic lateral pelvic node dissection. (**a**) Pelvic node dissection commences from common iliac vessels and then between external and internal iliac vessels to enter the obturator fossa. Ext Iliac A, external iliac artery; Ext Iliac V, external iliac vein; Int Iliac A, internal iliac artery. (**b**) A double-fenestrated grasper with jaws opened to retract the ureter, superior vesical artery, and external iliac vessels out of the targeted area. Ext Iliac V, external iliac vein; Int Iliac A, internal iliac artery; Sup Vesical A, superior vesical artery; Obturator N, obturator nerve; Hypogastric N, hypogastric nerve. (**c**) En bloc resection of lateral pelvic nodes is recommended, if possible. LPN, lateral pelvic node. (**d**) All lymphoareolar tissues were cleared leaving autonomic nerves and pelvic vessels intact. Ext Iliac A, external iliac artery; Ext Iliac V, external iliac vein; Int Iliac A, internal iliac artery; Sup Vesical A, superior vesical artery; Obturator N, obturator nerve; Hypogastric N, hypogastric nerve

7.7.2 Results of Robotic LPND

To our knowledge, the only paper published thus far on robotic LPND is our own preliminary study [19]. Thus, we will review our data only, including as yet unpublished data. To date, we have performed robotic TME + LPND in 18 patients with rectal cancer (unpublished). Our current indication for robotic LPND is persistent enlargement of LPN, even after preoperative CRT. Subsequently, a total of eight patients underwent preoperative CRT which was completed 8 weeks before surgery. All procedures were finished without conversion to either laparoscopic or open surgery. The mean height of the tumor was 4 cm from the anal verge. The mean time of operation and LPND were 272.5 (170–350) and 38 (20–51) min, respectively. The mean number of lateral lymph nodes harvested was 4.1 (range, 1 to 13). Three patients (38 %) were found to have lymph node metastases. Postoperative mortality and morbidity were 0 % and 25 %, respectively, but there was no LPND-related morbidity. The mean hospital stay was 7.5 (5–12) days. During a follow-up period of 24 months, local and distant relapse occurred in one patient (12.5 %) for each pattern of metastasis.

7.8 Discussion

We selected as candidates for LPND any patients with LPN larger than 5 mm in diameter, as shown on preoperative pelvic MRI, or any size with fluorine-18-fluorodeoxyglucose (FDG) uptake on PET-CT scan that were seen preoperatively. Those patients then underwent a long course of CRT, followed by reevaluation of LPN status just before surgery. Although our present study on robotic LPND reported only 38 % positivity of LPN, due to the small sample size, this double-filtering system increased the positive rate of LPN to over 56–71 %, even after CRT [16–18].

There are several important strategies to be discussed: first, the extent of LPND (total LPND vs limited LPND and ipsilateral vs bilateral LPND) and second, the neurovascular combined LPN resection or lymphoareolar dissection only. The Japanese group recommends that the external iliac group is not indicated for routine LPND unless metastatic nodes are suspected in that area [20]. The reason for this is that most common metastatic areas of LPN are found along the internal iliac vessels and obturator fossa. With regard to routine bilateral LPND, as many Japanese surgeons advocate [6, 7, 22, 23, 25, 26, 39], there is little evidence to support the notion that bilateral dissection is better than unilateral LPND if, clinically, only one side is suspected. As we previously experienced (unpublished), all lateral pelvic recurrences after LPND were presented on the side of positive LPN preoperatively, rather than on the untouched side of the pelvic wall. The Japanese group also recommends selective en bloc resection of LPN sacrificing branches of internal iliac vessels when therapeutic LPND is needed. In other cases, nerve- and vessel-preserving LPND is acceptable for prophylactic LPND in patients who do not have enlarged LPN pre- or intraoperatively [22].

As described previously, the role of the robot in LPND has not been well studied. After installation of a surgical robot at our institute, we recommended the robotic approach for patients who were indicated for minimally invasive LPND. This was due to the fact that robotic LPND appears to be more effective than the laparoscopic approach, as indicated by shorter operative times (272 min) and less bleeding (47.5 mL) as compared to our laparoscopic series showing 310 min and 188 mL, respectively. Additional advantages included the surgeon's ability to create the best surgical field by controlling the camera and three instruments and coordinating traction and counter-traction. Endo-wristed instruments also make it easier for the surgeon to dissect LPN in narrow confined areas, resulting in minimal hemorrhaging and precise nerve-sparing. These findings become even more prominent when compared to those of open surgery, even at large volume centers in

Japan. Finally, while, in general, the use of three-dimensional vision does not appear to be a big advantage to the experienced laparoscopic surgeon, it is one of the distinctive features of a surgical robot. For LPND, three-dimensional vision enables the surgeon to easily dissect LPNs that are entangled in networks of vessels and nerves. It is also worth noting that while using a single-incision access port, we found some usefulness for the multipurpose port in protecting the wound and thereby saving an additional assistant port as a route for stapling and retrieving the specimen, as well as for creating protective ileostomy if required.

Today, the use of indocyanine green (ICG) fluorescence imaging technology, combined with robotic infrared optics, has piqued the surgeons' interest in applying this technique to secure the blood supply of the resected bowel and to identify hidden lymph nodes [40–42]. In fact, this could play an important role in robotic LPND in the near future.

Overall, we find that the robotic approach for LPND following TME is technically feasible and safe. Robotic LPND can be one of the best options for the selected patient with advanced lower rectal cancer involving LPN.

7.9 Conclusions

Although many debates and controversies have been ongoing, metastasis of LPN is one of the major causes of local failure following surgery, and sterilization of positive LPN by either preoperative CRT or LPND may be beneficial to patients with lower rectal cancer. Still, it is clear that both modalities have limitations; thus, tailored treatment, or a combination of these two methods, might be the most reasonable alternative solution. In order to increase the accuracy of preoperative diagnostic modalities for selecting patients suitable to undergo LPND, standardization of diagnostic criteria is needed. Minimally invasive surgery, including the robotic approach for these selective situations, is both feasible and effective. Finally, large-scale clinical trials should be undertaken in order to prove the efficacy of robotic LPND.

Acknowledgments Responsibility to correspondence and study proposal are attributed to Gyu-Seog Choi. The study was not conducted under commercial sponsorship or grant. The author declares no conflict of interest.

References

1. Miles WE (1925) The spread of cancer of the rectum. Lancet 205:1218–1219
2. Coller FA, Kay EB, MacIntyre RS (1940) Regional lymphatic metastasis of carcinoma of the rectum. Surgery 8:294–311
3. Senba Y (1927) An anatomical study of lymphatic system of the rectum (in Japan). J Hukuoka Med Coll 20:1213–1268
4. Kuru M (1940) Cancer of the rectum (in Japanese). J Jpn Surg Soc 41:832–877

5. Hojo K (1986) Surgery of far-advanced colorectal cancer–extension of surgical indications and its results. Gan To Kagaku Ryoho 13(7):2282–2290
6. Sugihara K, Morya Y, Akasu T et al (1996) Pelvic autonomic nerve preservation for patients with rectal carcinoma. Oncologic and functional outcome. Cancer 78:1871–1880
7. Morya Y, Sugihara K, Akasu T et al (1997) Importance of extended lymphadenectomy with lateral node dissection for advanced lower rectal cancer. World J Surg 21:728–732
8. Swedish Rectal Cancer Trial (1997) Improved survival with preoperative radiotherapy in resectable rectal cancer. N Engl J Med 366(14):980–987
9. Kapiteijn E, Marijnen CAM, Nagtegaal ID et al (2001) Preoperative radiotherapy combined with total mesorectal excision for resectable rectal cancer. N Engl J Med 345(9):638–646
10. Sauer R, Becker H, Hohenberger W et al (2004) Preoperative versus postoperative chemoradiotherapy or rectal cancer. N Engl J Med 351:1731–1740
11. Watanabe T, Itabashi M, Shimada Y et al (2012) Japanese society for cancer of the colon and rectum (JSCCR) guidelines 2010 for the treatment of colorectal cancer. Int J Clin Oncol 17:1–29
12. Park IJ, Choi GS, Lim KH et al (2009) Laparoscopic resection of extraperitoneal rectal cancer: a comparative analysis with open resection. Surg Endosc 23(8):1818–1824
13. Jayne DG, Guillou PJ, Thorpe H et al (2007) Randomized trial of laparoscopic-assisted resection of colorectal carcinoma: 3-year results of the UK MRC CLASICC trial group. J Clin Oncol 25(21):3061–3068
14. van der Pas MH, Haglind E, Cuesta MA et al (2013) Laparoscopic versus open surgery for rectal cancer (COLOR II): short-term outcomes of a randomised, phase 3 trial. Lancet Oncol 14(3):210–218
15. Kang SB, Park JW, Jeong SY et al (2010) Open versus laparoscopic surgery for mid or low rectal cancer after neoadjuvant chemoradiotherapy (COREAN trial): short-term outcomes of an open-label randomised controlled trial. Lancet Oncol 11(7):637–645
16. Konishi T, Kuroyanagi H, Oya M et al (2011) Multimedia article. Lateral lymph node dissection with preoperative chemoradiation for locally advanced lower rectal cancer through a laparoscopic approach. Surg Endosc 25:2358–2359
17. Liang JT (2011) Technical feasibility of laparoscopic lateral pelvic node dissection for patients with low rectal cancer after concurrent chemoradiotherapy. Ann Surg Oncol 18(1):153–159
18. Park JS, Choi GS, Lim KH et al (2011) Laparoscopic extended lateral pelvic node dissection following total mesorectal excision for advanced rectal cancer: initial clinical experience. Surg Endosc 25:3322–3329
19. Park JA, Choi GS, Park JS et al (2012) Initial clinical experience with robotic lateral pelvic lymph node dissection for advanced rectal cancer. J Korean Soc Coloproctol 28(5):265–270
20. Kobayashi H, Mochizuki H, Kato T et al (2009) Outcomes of surgery alone for lower rectal cancer with and without pelvic sidewall dissection. Dis Colon Rectum 52:567–576
21. Akiyoshi T, Watanabe T, Ueno M (2012) Is lateral pelvic lymph node dissection no longer necessary for low rectal cancer after neoadjuvant therapy and TME to reduce local recurrence? J Gastrointest Surg 16:2341–2342
22. Fujita S, Akasu T, Mizusawa J et al (2012) Postoperative morbidity and mortality after mesorectal excision with and without lateral lymph node dissection for clinical stage II or stage III lower rectal cancer (JCOG0212): results from a multicentre, randomised controlled, non-inferiority trial. Lancet Oncol 13:616–621
23. Fujita S, Yamamoto S, Akasu T et al (2003) Lateral pelvic lymph node dissection for advanced lower rectal cancer. Br J Surg 90:1580–1585
24. Watanabe T, Tsurita G, Muto T et al (2002) Extended lymphadenectomy and preoperative radiotherapy for lower rectal cancers. Surgery 132:27–33
25. Ueno M, Oya M, Azekura K et al (2005) Incidence and prognostic significance of lateral lymph node metastasis in patients with advanced low rectal cancer. Br J Surg 92:756–763
26. Yano H, Moran BJ (2008) The incidence of lateral pelvic side-wall nodal involvement in low rectal cancer may be similar in Japan and the West. Br J Surg 95:33–49

27. Akasu T, Iinuma G, Takawa M et al (2009) Accuracy of high-resolution magnetic resonance imaging in preoperative staging of rectal cancer. Ann Surg Oncol 16:2787–2794
28. Yano H, Saito Y, Takeshita E et al (2007) Prediction of lateral pelvic node involvement in low rectal cancer by conventional computed tomography. Br J Surg 94:1014–1019
29. Arii K, Takifuji K, Yokoyama S et al (2006) Preoperative evaluation of pelvic lateral lymph node of patients with lower rectal cancer: comparison study of MR imaging and CT in 53 patients. Langenbecks Arch Surg 391:449–454
30. Syk E, Torkzad MR, Blomqvist L et al (2006) Radiological findings do not support lateral residual tumour as a major cause of local recurrence of rectal cancer. Br J Surg 93:113–119
31. Edge SB et al (2010) 7th edition of AJCC cancer staging handbook. Springer New York Dordrecht Heidelberg London
32. Kim TH, Jeong SY, Choi DH et al (2008) Lateral lymph node metastasis is a major cause of locoregional recurrence in rectal cancer treated with preoperative chemoradiotherapy and curative resection. Ann Surg Oncol 15:729–737
33. Enker WE, Thaler HT, Cranor ML et al (1995) Total mesorectal excision in the operative treatment of carcinoma of the rectum. J Am Coll Surg 181:335–346
34. Akasu T, Sugihara K, Moriya Y (2009) Male urinary and sexual functions after mesorectal excision alone or in combination with extended lateral pelvic lymph node dissection for rectal cancer. Ann Surg Oncol 16:2779–2786
35. Nishizawa Y, Ito M, Saito N et al (2011) Male sexual dysfunction after rectal cancer surgery. Int J Colorectal Dis 26:1541–1548
36. Georgiou P, Tan E, Gouvas N et al (2009) Extended lymphadenectomy versus conventional surgery for rectal cancer: a meta-analysis. Lancet Oncol 10:1053–1062
37. Kusters M, Beets GL, van de Velde CJ et al (2009) A comparison between the treatment of low rectal cancer in Japan and the Netherlands, focusing on the patterns of local recurrence. Ann Surg 249:229–235
38. Kim JC, Takahashi K, Yu CS et al (2007) Comparative outcome between chemoradiotherapy and lateral pelvic lymph node dissection following total mesorectal excision in rectal cancer. Ann Surg 246:754–762
39. Sugihara K, Kobayashi H, Kato T et al (2006) Indication and benefit of pelvic sidewall dissection for rectal cancer. Dis Colon Rectum 49:1663–1672
40. Jafari MD, Lee KH, Halabi WJ et al (2013) The use of indocyanine green fluorescence to assess anastomotic perfusion during robotic assisted laparoscopic rectal surgery. Surg Endosc 27(8):3003–3008
41. Holloway RW, Bravo RA, Rakowski JA et al (2012) Detection of sentinel lymph nodes in patients with endometrial cancer undergoing robotic-assisted staging: a comparison of colorimetric and fluorescence imaging. Gynecol Oncol 126(1):25–29
42. Rossi EC, Ivanova A, Boggess JF (2012) Robotically assisted fluorescence-guided lymph node mapping with ICG for gynecologic malignancies: a feasibility study. Gynecol Oncol 124(1):78–82

Cardiac Surgery: Overview

Go Watanabe

8.1 Introduction

The significant advantages of minimizing surgical trauma, such as reduced pain, shorter hospital stays, faster return to normal activities, and improved cosmesis, have resulted in the development of minimally invasive surgery [1]. Until recently, various difficulties associated with endoscopic approaches had stalled similar progress in the field of cardiac surgery. However, robotic technology overcame the difficulties associated with conventional endoscopic surgery and has made possible a new approach to minimally invasive cardiac surgery (MICS).

The application of robot-assisted coronary surgery ranges from internal mammary artery (IMA) harvesting with hand-sewn anastomoses to totally endoscopic coronary artery bypass grafting (TECAB) either on- or off-pump. The bilateral IMA can be harvested with the aid of a surgical robot and then multivessel bypass grafting can follow. Srivastava calls such robot-assisted minimally invasive direct coronary artery bypass grafting (MIDCAB) "ThoraCAB" [2]. Surgical robots can not only endoscopically harvest the IMA but they can also anastomose the coronary artery in TECAB.

On the other hand, closed-chest cardiopulmonary bypass (CPB) and cardioplegic arrest have stimulated the development of MICS via a small thoracotomy [3] and this has now become universal, especially to treat mitral valve defects and congenital structural heart diseases. Endoscopic techniques are also required for MICS, but conventional endoscopic instrumentation lacks the dexterity required for delicate cardiac surgical procedures, and the loss of depth perception caused by two-dimensional monitors further increases operative obstacles.

G. Watanabe (✉)
Department of General and Cardiothoracic Surgery, Kanazawa University, 13-1 Takaramachi, Kanazawa, Ishikawa 920-8641, Japan
e-mail: watago6633@gmail.com

Surgical robots have been developed to enhance surgical ability and precision and to repair structural heart conditions, including mitral valve plasty (MVP), atrial septal defect (ASD) closure, cardiac tumor resection, ThoraCAB, and TECAB. The Food and Drug Administration (FDA) cleared the da Vinci surgical system in 2000 for use in adult and pediatric urological, general, and gynecological laparoscopic surgeries, general non-cardiovascular thoracoscopic surgeries, and thoracoscopy-assisted cardiotomy procedures. The FDA also approved the da Vinci surgical system for use in coronary anastomosis during cardiac revascularization together with an adjunctive mediastinotomy in 2004 [4]. Over 1,700 robotic cardiac operations per year currently proceed in the USA and the numbers are increasing at an annual rate of about 25 % [5]. The most common applications in cardiac surgery are MVP and endoscopic coronary artery bypass grafting (CABG).

8.2 Robotic Surgery for Ischemic Heart Disease

8.2.1 ThoraCAB

The short-term patency rates of off-pump coronary artery bypass grafting (OPCAB) and CABG using CPB are similar, but OPCAB is associated with a reduced postoperative hospital stay, less demand for blood and blood components, and an earlier return to normal activities [6, 7]. MIDCAB through a left lateral thoracotomy without CPB confers all the benefits of OPCAB while avoiding morbidity caused by a median sternotomy. Thoracoscopic harvesting of the IMA avoids the hazards of conventional MIDCAB, and endoscopic IMA takedown has been regularly described since the 1990s [8]. Robotic IMA harvesting does not require a long incision or excessive opening of a thoracotomy and subsequent multivessel MIDCAB can proceed because the bilateral IMA can be harvested. ThoraCAB is thus a superlative CABG technique. Srivastava has implemented the largest reported single-institution series, with 200 patients undergoing robot-assisted bilateral IMA harvesting and off-pump CABG via a mini-thoracotomy [9].

8.2.2 TECAB

Watanabe et al. reported the first totally endoscopic CABG on a beating heart in 1999 [10], in which the left IMA was totally endoscopically harvested and anastomosed to the left anterior descending (LAD) using a customized suction endoscopic stabilizer that enabled immobilization of the anterior wall of the left ventricle through a thoracoport in two patients (Fig. 8.1). This procedure, which did not use a surgical robot, required a very advanced skill level. Stephenson et al. originally described 25 endoscopic coronary anastomoses of the coronary artery in 1998 using isolated porcine hearts in a reproduced human anatomical orientation and rib cage [11]. They performed a continuous end-to-side anastomosis between the harvested right coronary artery and the LAD coronary artery using the

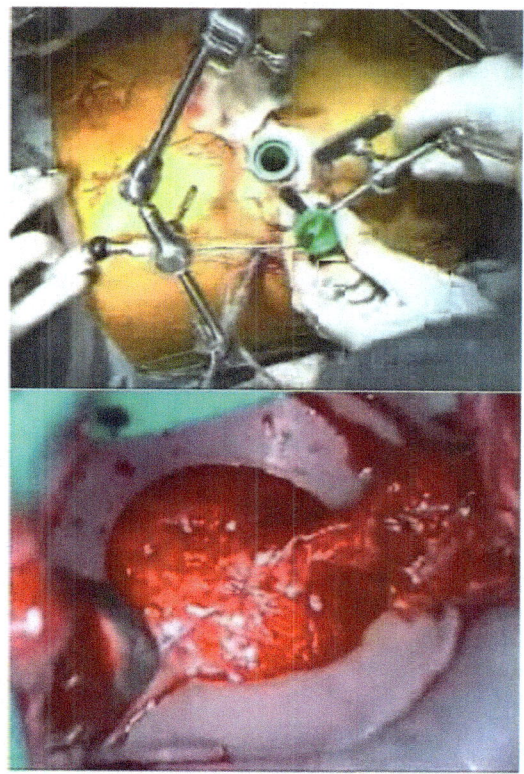

Fig. 8.1 Totally endoscopic coronary artery bypass grafting using endoscopic stabilizer without surgical robot

ZEUS system (Computer Motion) and a customized 6-cm double-armed 7-0 polytetrafluoroethylene suture. Loulmet et al. applied the first robotic TECAB in humans in 1998 [12]. They harvested and anastomosed the left IMA to the LAD using the first-generation da Vinci surgical system (Intuitive Surgical, Sunnyvale, CA, USA) in two men with cardiac arrest. Falk described the first off-pump robotic TECAB using an endoscopic stabilizing device in 2000 [13].

A port access stabilizer was required to achieve TECAB, and thus an EndoWrist stabilizer (Intuitive Surgical, Sunnyvale, CA, USA) was mounted on the fourth arm of the da Vinci surgical system (Fig. 8.2). This suction-type endostabilizer gives the console surgeon complete control, and these have led to highly complex endoscopic procedures such as triple and quadruple CABG being proceeding on arrested and beating hearts.

Srivastava et al. developed a technique for anastomosis during beating heart TECAB using U-clips (Medtronic. Minneapolis, MN, USA) [14] (Fig. 8.3). Robotically achieved interrupted coronary anastomosis also reduced the possibility of purse-stringing continuous sutures and helped to overcome the lack of tactile feedback inherent with the da Vinci surgical system. Intravascular ultrasonography showed that anastomosis is more compliant when performed in this manner with

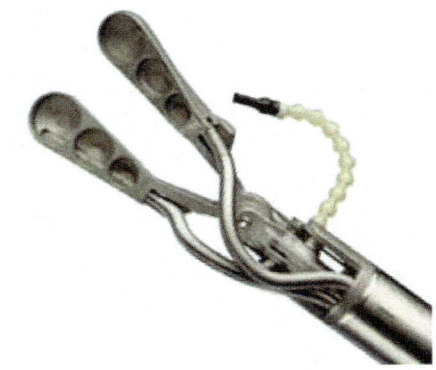

Fig. 8.2 EndoWrist stabilizer (from Intuitive Surgical's website)

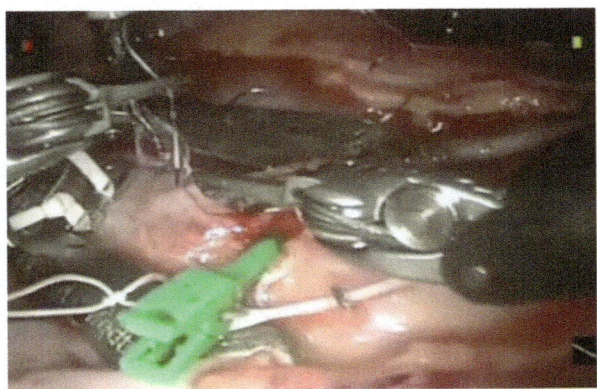

Fig. 8.3 Coronary anastomosis using U-clips in TECAB

continuous sutures than with running sutures [15]. However, U-clips are not universally available. On the other hand, Bonatti et al. reported 80 and 95 % success and safety rates, respectively, during a 10-year multicenter application of TECAB procedures in 500 patients. They preferentially applied arrested heart TECAB with cannulation of the femoral vessels, a balloon-tipped device (Cardiovation, Edwards Lifesciences Inc., Irvine, CA, USA or Estech, San Ramon, CA, USA) for aortic endo-occlusion [16], and anastomosis of the coronary artery using running 7-0 polypropylene sutures. Balkhy et al. used coronary anastomotic connectors in beating heart TECAB [17]. The C-Port Flex A distal anastomotic device (Cardica, Redwood City, CA, USA) was approved for use in the USA in 2005 after a multicenter European trial had shown >95 % vein graft patency at 6 months [18]. The C-Port device creates an end-to-side anastomosis using multiple interrupted stainless-steel clips (Fig. 8.4). The flexible shaft of the C-Port device allows its introduction through a port and facilitates a truly endoscopic approach to coronary bypass. They concluded that the C-Port device leads to a safe and reproducible robotic endoscopic single and multivessel coronary bypass under the beating heart with excellent short-term and midterm outcomes.

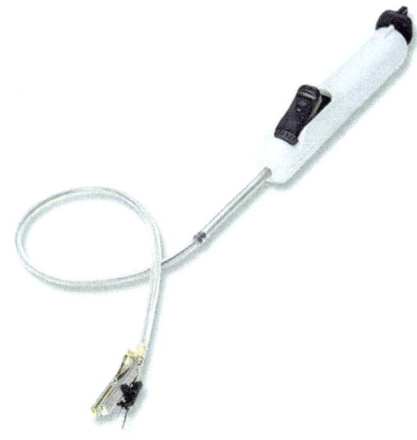

Fig. 8.4 C-Port Flex A distal anastomotic device (from Cardica's website)

8.3 Hybrid Procedure

The indications for CABG and percutaneous coronary intervention (PCI) for multivessel coronary artery disease remain controversial [19, 20]. Hybrid revascularization combines minimally invasive coronary artery bypass, such as ThoraCAB and TECAB, with PCI of other stenosed arteries; integrating these two procedures into one therapeutic modality aims to provide patients with the benefits of each successive technique in the least invasive way. This approach is likely to become more popular, particularly with advances in robotic instrumentation. The survival benefit of the left IMA for ostial or complex lesions of the LAD has been established [21]. Bonatti et al. described the feasibility and safety of simultaneous hybrid coronary revascularization [22, 23]. Srivastava et al. also reported that beating heart TECAB was safe, effective, and less invasive and also offered the option of the hybrid procedure with excellent early clinical and graft patency for selected patients with single and multivessel coronary artery disease [24, 25].

8.4 Robotic Surgery for Structural Heart Disease

8.4.1 Mitral Valve Surgery

Carpentier performed the first robotic MVP using an early prototype of the da Vinci surgical system in May 1998 [26]. and Mohr performed the first coronary anastomosis and repaired five mitral valves using the system one week later [27]. Grossi et al. partially repaired a mitral valve using the ZEUS system [28] and Chitwood performed the first complete da Vinci MVP in North America 4 days later in May 2000 [29].

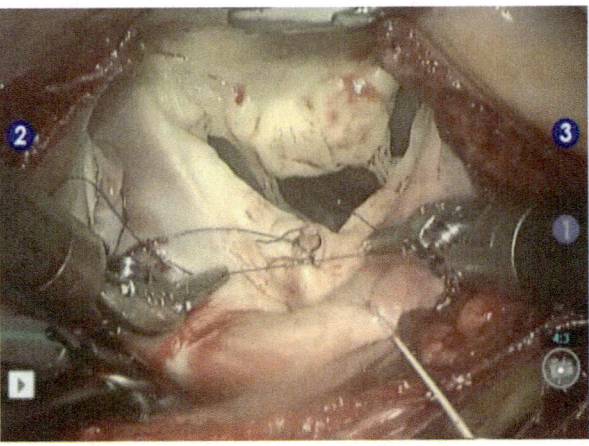

Fig. 8.5 Robot-assisted mitral valve plasty

Two subsequent studies demonstrated that robotic mitral valve surgery is safe, the short-term results are excellent, and the midterm durability is good [30, 31]. The FDA approved the da Vinci surgical system for mitral valve surgery and ASD repair in November 2002. Mitral valve surgery was accomplished through the same small thoracotomy incisions as the MICS procedure, since the surgical robot allowed the surgeons to complete complex maneuvers. The robotic system is now frequently applied to mitral valve surgery that customarily proceeds through a small thoracotomy, and robot-assisted totally endoscopic MVP has recently become popular [32] (Fig. 8.5).

Suri et al. evaluated the postoperative quality-of-life indices among asymptomatic or minimally symptomatic patients after undergoing isolated MVP for mitral valve regurgitation and concluded that those who were treated using robot-assisted MVP returned to work slightly sooner than those who were treated using a conventional transsternotomy procedure [33]. Cohn et al. reported that a minimally invasive approach was associated with a reduced need for red blood cell transfusion, greater patient satisfaction, and a 20 % reduction in costs compared with the conventional approach [34].

8.4.2 Surgery for Congenital Heart Disease

Le Bret et al. concluded that surgical durations are comparable between robot-assisted patent ductus arteriosus (PDA) closure using the ZEUS system and videothoracoscopic techniques [35]. ASD closure using direct suture repair or patches has also been accomplished with robotics [36]. Secundum ASD or patent foramen ovale with or without mitral valve regurgitation should also be addressable with surgical robots (Fig. 8.6) and sinus venosus ASD has been also repaired in this manner. Gao et al. found that on-pump ASD repairs of the beating heart using the da Vinci surgical system without cross-clamping the aorta was feasible, safe, and

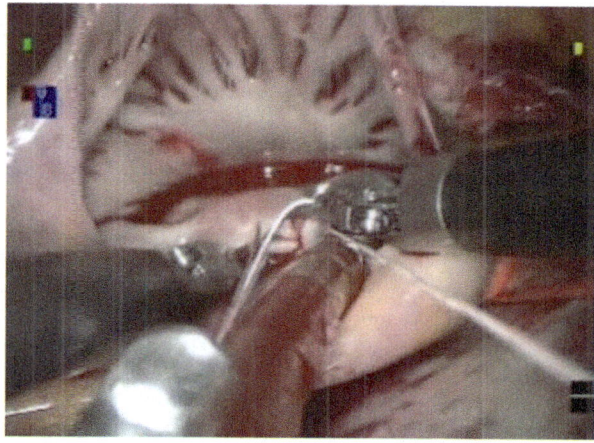

Fig. 8.6 Robot-assisted atrial septal defect closure

effective [37]. Gao et al. also described robot-assisted totally endoscopic repair of a ventricular septal defect using a dynamic atrial retractor (Intuitive Surgical) to elevate the anterior leaflet of the tricuspid valve.

References

1. Modi P, Hassan A, Chitwood WR Jr (2008) Minimally invasive mitral valve surgery: a systematic review and meta-analysis. Eur J Cardiothorac Surg 34:943–952
2. Srivastava S, Gadasalli S, Agusala M, Kolluru R, Naidu J, Shroff M, Barrera R, Quismundo S, Srivastava V (2006) Use of bilateral internal thoracic arteries in CABG through lateral thoracotomy with robotic assistance in 150 patients. Ann Thorac Surg 81:800–806
3. Iribarne A, Easterwood R, Chan EY, Yang J, Soni L, Russo MJ, Smith CR, Argenziano M (2011) The golden age of minimally invasive cardiothoracic surgery: current and future perspectives. Future Cardiol 7:333–746
4. Intuitive Surgical (2013) Surgical specialties – regulatory clearance. http://www.intuitivesurgical.com/specialties/regulatory-clearance.html. Accessed 21 Feb 2013
5. Robicsek F (2008) Robotic cardiac surgery: time told! J Thorac Cardiovasc Surg 135:243–246
6. Cooley DA (2000) Beating-heart surgery for coronary revascularization: is it the most important development since the introduction of the heart-lung machine? Ann Thorac Surg 70:1779–1781
7. Contini M, Iacò A, Iovino T, Teodori G, Di Giammarco G, Mazzei V, Commodo M, Calafiore AM (1999) Current results in off pump surgery. Eur J Cardiothorac Surg 16:69–72
8. Watanabe G, Misaki T, Kotoh K, Yamashita A, Ueyama K (1998) Bilateral thoracoscopic minimally invasive direct coronary artery bypass grafting using internal thoracic arteries. Ann Thorac Surg 65:1673–1675
9. Srivastava SP, Patel KN, Skantharaja R, Barrera R, Nanayakkara D, Srivastava V (2003) Off-pump complete revascularization through a left lateral thoracotomy (ThoraCAB): the first 200 cases. Ann Thorac Surg 76:46–49
10. Watanabe G, Takahashi M, Misaki T, Kotoh K, Doi Y (1999) Beating-heart endoscopic coronary artery surgery. Lancet 354:2131–2132
11. Stephenson ER Jr, Sankholkar S, Ducko CT, Damiano RJ Jr (1998) Robotically assisted microsurgery for endoscopic coronary artery bypass grafting. Ann Thorac Surg 66:1064–1067

12. Loulmet D, Carpentier A, d' Attelis N et al (1999) Endoscopic coronary artery bypass grafting with the aid of computer-assisted instruments. J Thorac Cardiovasc Surg 48:4–10
13. Falk V, Diegeler A, Walther T, Banusch J, Brucerius J, Raumans J, Autschbach R, Mohr FW (2000) Total endoscopic computer enhanced coronary artery bypass grafting. Eur J Cardiothorac Surg 17:38–45
14. Srivastava S, Gadasalli S, Agusala M, Kolluru R, Barrera R, Quismundo S, Kreaden U, Jeevanandam V (2010) Beating heart totally endoscopic coronary artery bypass. Ann Thorac Surg 89:1873–1880
15. Hamman B, White C (2004) Interrupted distal anastomosis: the interrupted "porcupine" technique. Ann Thorac Surg 78:722–724
16. Schachner T, Bonaros N, Wiedemann D, Weidinger F, Feuchtner G, Friedrich G, Laufer G, Bonatti J (2009) Training surgeons to perform robotically assisted totally endoscopic coronary surgery. Ann Thorac Surg 88:523–527
17. Balkhy HH, Wann LS, Arnsdorf SE, Maciolek K (2009) Long term patency evaluation of the cardica c-port distal anastomotic device in coronary bypass grafting: initial experience in 91 grafts. Innovations 4:158
18. Matschke KE, Gummert JF, Demertzis S et al (2005) The Cardica C-Port system: clinical and angiographic evaluation of a new device for automated, compliant distal anastomoses in coronary artery bypass grafting surgery—a multicenter prospective clinical trial. J Thorac Cardiovasc Surg 130:1645–1652
19. Takayama T, Hiro T, Hirayama A (2010) Is angioplasty able to become the gold standard of treatment beyond bypass surgery for patients with multivessel coronary artery disease? Therapeutic strategies for 3-vessel coronary artery disease: OPCAB vs PCI (PCI-Side). Circ J 74:2744–2749
20. Nishimi M, Tashiro T (2010) Off-pump coronary artery bypass vs percutaneous coronary intervention. Therapeutic strategies for 3-vessel coronary artery disease: OPCAB vs PCI (PCI-Side). Circ J 74:2750–2757
21. Gao C, Yang M, Wu Y, Wang G, Xiao C, Liu H, Lu C (2009) Hybrid coronary revascularization by endoscopic robotic coronary artery bypass grafting on beating heart and stent placement. Ann Thorac Surg 87:737–741
22. Bonatti JO, Zimrin D, Lehr EJ, Vesely M, Kon ZN, Wehman B, de Biasi AR, Hofauer B, Weidinger F, Schachner T, Bonaros N, Friedrich G (2012) Hybrid coronary revascularization using robotic totally endoscopic surgery: perioperative outcomes and 5-year results. Ann Thorac Surg 94:1920–1926, discussion 1926
23. Bonatti J, Lehr E, Vesely MR, Friedrich G, Bonaros N, Zimrin D (2010) Hybrid coronary revascularization: which patients? When? How? Curr Opin Cardiol 25:568–574
24. Srivastava S, Barrera R, Quismundo S (2012) One hundred sixty-four consecutive beating heart totally endoscopic coronary artery bypass cases without intraoperative conversion. Ann Thorac Surg 94:1463–1468
25. Srivastava S, Gadasalli S, Tijerina O, Barrera R, Quismundo S, Srivastava V (2006) Planned simultaneous beating-heart totally endoscopic coronary artery bypass (TECAB) and percutaneous intervention in a single operative setting. Innovations 1:239–242
26. Carpentier A, Loulmet D, Aupecle B, Kieffer JP, Tournay D, Guibourt P, Fiemeyer A, Meleard D, Richomme P (1998) Cardon C [Computer assisted open heart surgery. First case operated on with success]. CR Acad Sci III 321:437–442
27. Mohr FW, Falk V, Diegeler A, Autschback R (1999) Computer-enhanced coronary artery bypass surgery. J Thorac Cardiovasc Surg 117:1212–1214
28. Grossi EA, Lapietra A, Applebaum RM, Ribakove GH, Galloway AC, Baumann FG, Ursomanno P, Steinberg BM, Colvin SB (2000) Case report of robotic instrument-enhanced mitral valve surgery. J Thorac Cardiovasc Surg 120:1169–1171
29. Chitwood WR Jr, Nifong LW, Elbeery JE, Chapman WH, Albrecht R, Kimitral V, Young JA (2000) Robotic mitral valve repair: trapezoidal resection and prosthetic annuloplasty with the da vinci surgical system. J Thorac Cardiovasc Surg 120:1171–1172

30. Nifong LW, Chu VF, Bailey BM, Maziarz DM, Sorrell VL, Holbert D, Chitwood WR Jr (2003) Robotic mitral valve repair: experience with the da Vinci system. Ann Thorac Surg 75:438–442, discussion 43
31. Nifong LW, Chitwood WR, Pappas PS, Smith CR, Argenziano M, Starnes VA, Shah PM (2005) Robotic mitral valve surgery: a United States multicenter trial. J Thorac Cardiovasc Surg 129:1395–1404
32. Rodríguez E, Kypson AP, Moten SC, Nifong LW, Chitwood WR Jr (2006) Robotic mitral surgery at East Carolina University: a 6 year experience. Int J Med Robot 2:211–215
33. Suri RM, Antiel RM, Burkhart HM, Huebner M, Li Z, Eton DT, Topilsky T, Sarano ME, Schaff HV (2012) Quality of life after early mitral valve repair using conventional and robotic approaches. Ann Thorac Surg 93:761–769
34. Cohn LH, Adams DH, Couper GS, Bichell DP, Rosborough DM, Sears SP, Aranki SF (1997) Minimally invasive cardiac valve surgery improves patient satisfaction while reducing costs of cardiac valve replacement and repair. Ann Surg 226:421–426, discussion 427–428
35. Le Bret E, Papadatos S, Folliguet T, Carbognani D, Pétrie J, Aggoun Y, Batisse A, Bachet J, Laborde F (2002) Interruption of patent ductus arteriosus in children: robotically assisted versus videothoracoscopic surgery. J Thorac Cardiovasc Surg 123:973–976
36. Reichenspurner H, Boehm DH, Welz A et al (1998) 3-D-video- and robot-assisted minimally invasive ASD closure using the port-access techniques. Heart Surg Forum 1:104–106
37. Gao C, Yang M, Wang G, Wang J, Xiao C, Wu Y, Li J (2010) Totally endoscopic robotic atrial septal defect repair on the beating heart. Heart Surg Forum 13:155–158

Robotically Assisted Totally Endoscopic Coronary Artery Bypass Grafting

Johannes Bonatti, Stephanie Mick, Nikolaos Bonaros, Eric Lehr, Ravi Nair, and Tomislav Mihaljevic

9.1 Introduction

Totally endoscopic coronary artery bypass grafting (TECAB) can only be performed on a routine basis using robotic technology. Since the first reports of TECAB in the late 1990s significant technological and surgical progress has been made. Currently a third generation of surgical robots is available which offers differentiated procedure-specific instrumentation. Using this technology single, double, triple, and even quadruple coronary artery bypass grafting is now feasible.

The technique presented herein was developed by robotic heart surgery teams at the Innsbruck Medical University, the University of Maryland, the Swedish Hospital in Seattle, the Cleveland Clinic Main Campus, and the Cleveland Clinic Abu Dhabi using the da Vinci Si model (Intuitive Surgical, Sunnyvale CA, USA). We focus on indications, patient workup, surgical details, and postoperative care. Concerning results and general evaluation of the method the reader is referred to current review articles in the literature [1–3].

J. Bonatti, M.D. FETCS (✉) • R. Nair • T. Mihaljevic
Department of Cardiothoracic Surgery, Heart & Vascular Institute, Cleveland Clinic Abu Dhabi, Abu Dhabi, PO Box 112412, United Arab Emirates
e-mail: bonattj@clevelandclinicabudhabi.ae

S. Mick
Cleveland Clinic, Cleveland, OH, USA

N. Bonaros
Innsbruck Medical University, Innsbruck, Austria

E. Lehr
Swedish Hospital, Seattle, WA, USA

9.2 Indications and Contraindications

At the current stage of development any patient with single or multivessel coronary artery disease with a clear indication for surgical revascularization can be taken into consideration for TECAB. Still, proper patient selection is of utmost importance in this type of surgery, especially during the initial installation of a TECAB program. As a general principle the surgeon should choose low-risk patients during the implementation phase of robotic coronary artery bypass grafting at a given program. If hybrid coronary intervention is an option, it is advisable to give the hybrid approach preference to reduce TECAB complexity as compared to multivessel TECAB. The indication and surgical approach should be thoroughly discussed with the referring cardiologist, the patient, and the family.

During an institutional and surgeon's learning curve technical errors may happen which can usually be tolerated by patients without comorbidities but detrimental in patients with multiple comorbidities. The surgical team is also advised to stay away from acute and unstable patients in the early phase of program development. Robotic coronary bypass surgery (CABG) is essentially elective. Surgeons with little experience should start with single-vessel disease in patients without significant comorbidities.

Table 9.1 lists the main contraindications for TECAB. Special attention should be paid to patients with significant lung disease; such patients do not tolerate extended periods of single-lung ventilation. Intrathoracic space is limited in patients with enlarged hearts and technical challenges are likely. Redo operations are feasible, but takedown of adhesions is demonding and bleeding can be difficult to handle in the completely endoscopic setting. Generalized vasculopathy is a contraindication for femoral retrograde heart-lung machine perfusion and for use

Table 9.1 Contraindications for TECAB

Absolute
Cardiogenic shock and hemodynamic instability
Severely reduced lung function
Significantly enlarged hearts
Pulmonary hypertension
Chest deformities
Multimorbid patients with generalized vasculopathy
Very small, diffusely diseased and calcified target vessels in beating heart TECAB
Ascending aortic diameter > 3.8 mm and moderate/severe aortoiliac atherosclerosis in arrested heart TECAB using the endoballoon
Relative
Unstable patients on IABP
Significantly reduced left ventricular function
St. p. previous cardiac surgery
St. p. chest trauma
St. p. chest radiation

of the endoballoon. These patients should undergo beating heart TECAB and are a risk group in any type of coronary artery bypass grafting. Patients with very small diffusely diseased target vessels or intramyocardial target vessels should undergo the arrested heart version of the procedure.

9.3 Preoperative Evaluation

All patients should receive the same workup as is common practice in open CABG. Special attention should be paid to preoperative lung function and spirometry is mandatory. Our own experience has shown that an FEV1 of less than 2.5 l is a cutoff value. We have observed that under this level intraoperative technical difficulties related to space limitations and postoperative morbidity increase. Every patient must undergo a preoperative CT angiography of the chest, abdomen, and pelvis to assess for size of the heart, size of the pericardial fatpad, relation of the internal mammary arteries to the target vessels, intramyocardial course of target vessels, ascending aortic diameter, and grade of aortoiliac atherosclerosis. In our experience a distance of less than 25 mm from the left heart border to the chest wall due to reduced space can lead to surgical technical challenges due to limited working space.

9.4 Time-Out

Proper information about procedure details (planned target vessels and conduits, cannulation site, etc.) is key. The preoperative CT scan and the coronary angiogram should be displayed on screen in the operating room. Perfusion strategies must be discussed and it is important to have a last look at the intraoperative TEE screen. Previously undetected findings such as significant aortic arch atherosclerosis or valve disease may be detected. It is strongly recommended to use a preoperative checklist to ensure that all equipment (including all equipment for conversion to CABG if necessary) is available before start of the operation.

9.5 Anesthesia

Monitoring and the general conduct of anesthesia are the same as in open CABG through sternotomy. To gain space for instrumentation ipsilateral lung collapse is necessary. Therefore a double-lumen endotracheal tube or a bronchial blocker is inserted. R2 defibrillator patches are placed with care taken that adequate current flow is enabled and that they are placed in positions that still allow performance of a sternotomy. TEE is necessary throughout the whole procedure. An EndoVent and/or a percutaneous retrograde cardioplegia cannula is placed in cases of arrested heart TECAB.

9.6 Positioning, Prepping, and Draping

The patient is placed on the operating table in the supine position. The arms are tucked to the body and the left chest is slightly elevated using a subscapular pillow or towel roll. Prepping and draping is the same as for open CABG. All equipment for conversion to open CABG should be in the room at the start of the procedure. Participation of the whole team in this part of the procedure can speed up the whole TECAB process.

9.7 The Role of the Heart-Lung Machine in Robotic CABG

TECAB can be performed with and without use of cardiopulmonary bypass. The former version is usually called AH (arrested heart)-TECAB; the latter is commonly referred to as BH (beating heart)-TECAB. Our group performs both versions of the procedure and tailors the operation to the needs of the patient.

It is absolutely clear that many patients benefit from beating heart approaches and TECAB surgeons should develop familiarity with BH-TECAB. Endoscopic suturing, however, is technically more challenging than the arrested heart approach and surgeons are advised to perform on-pump operations with endo-cardioplegia first. If BH-TECAB is planned, we strongly discourage the use of peripheral cannulation and the heart-lung machine only in cases of technical difficulties. The worst-case scenario is intraoperative ventricular fibrillation and the necessity of resuscitation measures with the robot docked. Without prophylactic cannulation and the ability to initiate cardiopulmonary bypass, the situation can rapidly grow dire. Such situations have occurred and have destroyed emerging TECAB programs. It is therefore highly recommended to prophylactically cannulate the patient under controlled conditions so that a heart-lung machine run is available immediately. This strategy also allows one to gain significant additional space inside the chest by starting the pump and deflating both lungs. In some patients this is the only way to develop adequate space and hemodynamics to access the back wall of the heart.

Arrested heart TECAB on the other hand requires specific perfusion and cardioplegia skills. Remote access heart-lung machine perfusion and the use of ascending aortic balloon occlusion are technically challenging and require very careful patient selection. Femoral perfusion and endoballoon should only be used in patients without aortoiliac atherosclerosis. Approximately two thirds of patients currently eligible for TECAB fall into this category. Axillary antegrade perfusion and femoral insertion of the endoballoon is the best option for patients with moderate grades of aortoiliac atherosclerosis. Transthoracic clamping and direct aortic root cannulation for cardioplegia is an option but in its early stage of development. Challenges associated with this technique include transthoracic puncture of the ascending aorta and insertion of an appropriate catheter as well as endoscopic robotic control of bleeding after catheter removal.

Surgeons are advised to develop remote access perfusion techniques in other minimally invasive heart surgical procedures before they apply them in TECAB.

Introducing both robotic coronary surgery and advanced peripheral heart-lung machine techniques at the same time can be detrimental and should absolutely be avoided.

With the above measures in mind, we have found that both AH-TECAB and BH-TECAB can be performed safely and can become fascinating operations performed at a high comfort level.

9.8 Operative Technique

9.8.1 Port Placement

Correct insertion of the endoscopy ports is a key maneuver which significantly influences the success of the whole procedure. Port placement should therefore be performed by the most experienced team member. The surgeon should make sure that the ipsilateral lung is completely deflated before insertion of the first port which should be the camera port. A 12.5 mm port is used and inserted into the fifth intercostal space on the anterior axillary line. This port has to be placed very gently and cautiously so as to avoid injury to the intrathoracic organs. After insertion and removal of the trocar CO_2 is inflated at pressures of 8 mmHg. Under videoscopic vision with the 30-degree angled camera the left and right instrument ports are placed into the 3rd and 7th intercostal spaces slightly anterior to the camera port. The robotic system is then docked. During this phase the surgical team should be aware of a potential hemodynamic compromise by the CO_2 insufflation. CO_2 pressure can be lowered as needed. Communication with the anesthesia team is critical. If hemodynamic compromise develops during insufflation, the first corrective maneuver to be performed is to lower the CO_2 pressure rather than fluid or inotrope administration.

9.8.2 Internal Mammary Artery (IMA) Harvesting

This part of the procedure is done with the angled camera view up. The robotic electrocautery spatula on the right and a DeBakey forceps on the left are inserted into the instrument ports under camera guidance. Using low power levels (we use 15 W) on the electrocautery the endothoracic fascia is detached from the internal mammary artery (IMA) pedicle, giving the team a perfect view on the conduit. The IMA is harvested in skeletonized technique mostly by cauterizing side branches (Fig. 9.1). In general, most side branches can be cauterized with clips used for larger branches. The operator should use the cautery tip for dividing the adjacent tissue mechanically, i.e., by spatulation rather than tissue-burning maneuvers. After harvesting and heparinization the conduit is clipped distally and divided. It is then dropped into the left pleural space to allow autodilation. Both the left and the right IMA can be taken down using the above technique and with the same port

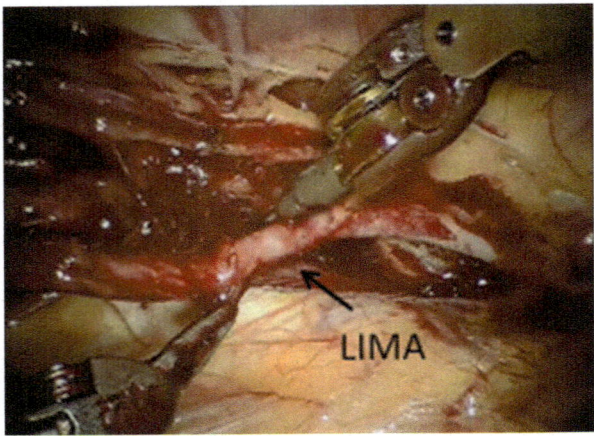

Fig. 9.1 The left internal mammary artery (LIMA) is harvested in skeletonized technique using robotic DeBakey forceps on the *left* and a robotic electrocautery spatula on the *right*

arrangement. To access the right IMA the retrosternal tissue is divided and the right pleura is entered. When bilateral conduits are used the right IMA is harvested before the left IMA.

9.8.3 Placement of the Assistance Port

In our experience the TECAB procedure is smoother and faster with the use of transthoracic assistance. A 5 mm assistance port is placed after IMA harvesting in the left parasternal region under scope visualization. This port allows insertion of material needed throughout the procedure such as bulldogs, suture material, silastic tapes, and suction tubing.

9.8.4 Removal of the Pericardial Fatpad and Pericardiotomy

This part of the operation is best done with the angled camera view down. To access the heart the pericardial fatpad is mobilized and dropped into the left chest. The best instrument combination for this is a robotic long-tip forceps on the left and electrocautery at 30 W on the right. For pericardiotomy we use the same instruments. The pericardium is incised slightly lateral to the right ventricular outflow tract. It is opened all the way down to the reflection of the pericardium. The incision is then taken laterally in the caudal and cranial part so that a pericardial flap is created which falls into the left pleural space. If the heart-lung machine is used the heart can be unloaded during this phase and fatpad removal as well as pericardiotomy are significantly easier to perform, especially in obese patients and patients with enlarged hearts.

9.8.5 Use of Cardiopulmonary Bypass

If there is no aortoiliac atherosclerosis on the preoperative CT angiography, femorofemoral heart-lung machine perfusion and the use of the endoaortic balloon are safe. Cannulation maneuvers are carried out under strict TEE guidance. The femoral vessels are exposed in the groin, usually on the left side. All cannulation maneuvers in these cases can be carried out while one team member is harvesting the IMA robotically. We place cannulae with the patient heparinized to an ACT of 300 s and add heparin to an ACT of 480 s shortly before the start of cardiopulmonary bypass. It is of great importance to ensure arterial distal leg perfusion and we therefore insert a distal perfusion cannula into the superficial femoral artery in all cases. Then a 21 or 23 F arterial perfusion cannula with a side arm for the endoballoon catheter is then inserted and connected to the heart-lung machine tubing. Likewise a 25 F venous drainage cannula is brought up into the right atrium and superior vena cava and connected to the heart-lung machine tubing as well. The aortic endoballoon catheter is inserted into the side arm of the arterial perfusion cannula and then advanced into the aortic root over a guidewire. The catheter is connected to the cardioplegia-vent line of the heart-lung machine and aortic root pressure and balloon pressure lines are connected to the monitoring devices. Once adequate ACT levels are confirmed, the heart-lung machine is started slowly. It is important to ensure that adequate venous drainage has been achieved and that a drop in systemic perfusion pressure is observed. Without ventricular ejections balloon placement is easier. The surgeon locates the endoballoon on an adequately visible TEE monitor and inflates the balloon. An injection of 6 mg of adenosine into the aortic root induces cardioplegia immediately and this is followed by infusion of cardioplegia into the aortic root. If a percutaneous retrograde cardioplegia catheter was placed into the coronary sinus, a usual protocol of ante- and retrograde infusion of cardioplegia can be followed. The patient is cooled to 35°c in single AH-TECAB and to 32°c in multivessel TECAB.

If mild to moderate aortoiliac atherosclerosis is present, we avoid arterial retroperfusion through the femoral artery and cannulate the left axillary artery. For anatomical access reasons this is best done before docking of the robotic arms. The vessel is exposed in the left infraclavicular region, clamped, and incised, and an 8 mm Dacron prosthesis side arm is sutured to the axillary artery. After proper deairing the side arm is connected to the heart-lung machine tubing. The aortic endoballoon in these cases is inserted through a separate 19 F cannula in the femoral artery.

Should the preoperative CT angiography show significant aortoiliac and general atherosclerosis we do not use the endoballoon at all. We operate these patients on the beating heart with prophylactic peripheral cannulation. The axillary artery is exposed and cannulated as described above. The venous drainage cannula is inserted from the groin in percutaneous or open fashion. An ACT level of 300 s is again used for cannulation. Before starting the anastomotic suturing on the beating heart the ACT is increased to above 480 s Using this strategy the pump can be started expeditiously at any time should significant technical difficulties occur.

9.8.6 Exposure of Target Vessels

For all work on the coronary targets we use a camera down view. The left anterior descending artery (LAD) with the port arrangements mentioned above can be visualized and accessed without difficulties. In beating heart TECAB and arrested heart cases with lateral target vessels the LAD can be moved into an easily accessible position using the robotic endostabilizer. The endostabilizer is brought in through a subcostal port inserted two fingerbreadths left lateral to the xiphoid angle. The subcostal port is docked to the fourth arm of the robotic system.

For exposure of the circumflex coronary artery system the endostabilizer is used as well. The da Vinci Si system allows that the operator steers the endostabilizer gently over the left ventricle. The lateral wall can be lifted up and obtuse marginal branches can be accessed. In beating heart TECAB this maneuver can lead to hemodynamic compromise and signs of ischemia. A supportive heart-lung machine run easily or addresses this problem.

We have recently developed a method to expose the right coronary artery system from the patient's left side. The endostabilizer is inserted through the left instrument port (a 12 mm port is necessary) and the left robotic instrument is inserted through the subcostal port. The acute margin can be lifted up in a way that the posterior descending artery and the posterolateral branch are well visible and accessible for anastomosis. It should be noted that thus far this technique has only been performed on the arrested heart. Care has to be taken not to cause injury to the right ventricular epimyocardium with the endostabilizer.

Once the target coronary artery is properly located and exposed the epicardium above the vessel is incised using robotic DeBakey forceps on the left and robotic Potts scissors on the right. This part of the procedure is probably the only one in which the surgeon has to adapt to the lack of tactile feedback during the learning curve. With time, however, full comfort level can be achieved.

9.8.7 Robotic Endoscopic Graft to Coronary Artery Anastomosis (General Technique)

The target vessel is incised using robotic DeBakey forceps on the left and robotic lancet beaver knife on the right. For anastomotic suturing, we take a 7/0 double-armed polypropylene suture, 7 cm in length. Bilateral robotic black diamond microforceps are used as needle drivers. The first stitch is inside-out on the back wall of the anastomosis close to the toe. The needle is then parked in the epicardium and we continue with the other needle suturing the whole back wall going inside-out on the graft and outside-in on the target vessel. The first three stitches are placed in a parachute technique and the graft is then brought towards the coronary artery wall. The operator gently pulls on both suture ends frequently to ensure adequate suture tension (Fig. 9.2). Suturing then continues around the heel of the anastomosis again suturing the graft inside-out and the target vessel in an outside-in fashion (Fig. 9.3). The needle is then parked in the epicardium and the previously used

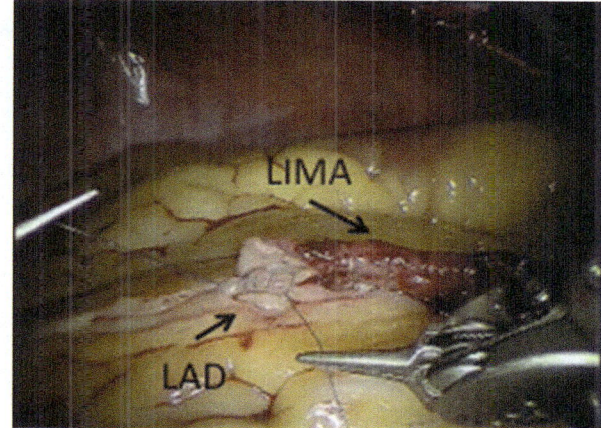

Fig. 9.2 The back wall of the anastomosis is sutured first. The surgeon pulls on both suture ends frequently in order to ensure adequate suture tension. *LIMA* left internal mammary artery, *LAD* left anterior descending artery

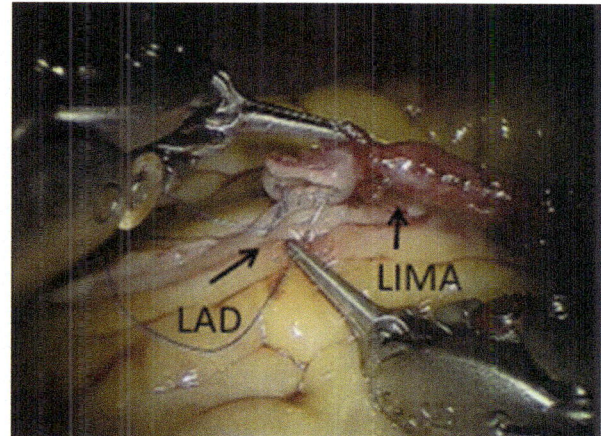

Fig. 9.3 The heel of the anastomosis is sutured next going outside-in on the target vessel and inside-out on the graft. *LIMA* left internal mammary artery, *LAD* left anterior descending artery

needle is used to suture the toe and the rest of the anterior wall of the anastomosis. An endoscopically completed left internal mammary artery (LIMA) to LAD bypass is shown in Fig. 9.4.

9.8.8 Anastomotic Suturing in Arrested Heart TECAB

The coronary artery can be incised with antegrade cardioplegia running. This reduces the risk of injury to the back wall. If there is backflow from the target vessel which prevents a clear view on the anastomotic interior the surgeon should liberally use silastic tapes to occlude the vessel. With the heart arrested using endocardioplegia the suturing comfort is usually very high. Gentle probing maneuvers at the toe and heel before completion of the anastomosis using microforceps can be

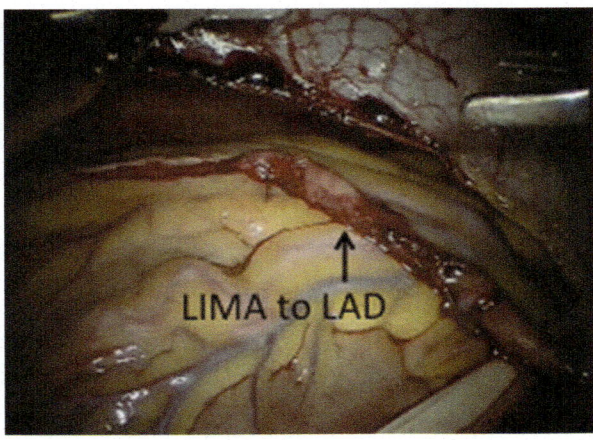

Fig. 9.4 View on the completed left internal mammary artery to left anterior descending artery (LIMA to LAD) bypass

performed safely. All foreign material should be removed from the chest before the aortic endoballoon is deflated. The heart may later on become hyperdynamic and these maneuvers will be difficult.

9.8.9 Anastomotic Suturing in Beating Heart TECAB

We place silastic tapes proximally and distally to the anastomotic site. Usually only the proximal one needs to be occluded. An intraluminal shunt is inserted into the distal target vessel and then advanced into the proximal target vessel. The general suturing is the same as in arrested heart TECAB. All stitches have to be carried out very gently so as to avoid injury to the target vessel wall. With time the surgeon will learn how to deal with the magnified bouncing operative field.

9.8.10 Special Aspects in Multivessel TECAB

For multivessel TECAB the development of sequential and Y-grafting techniques is necessary. Both internal mammary in situ grafts can be used as inflow. The contralateral IMA or a radial artery is available for the construction of Y-grafts. Another option is the use of an endoscopically harvested vein graft sutured to the left axillary artery. The techniques for endoscopic construction and placement of these bypass grafts were recently described in our report on the first successful quadruple bypass [3].

9.8.11 Intraoperative Quality Control

After completion of the anastomosis the bulldog clamp on the graft is removed. In the robotic endoscopic setting repair stitches due to the high magnification can be placed with very good overview if necessary. The endostabilizer is removed from the chest and an endoscopic transit time flowprobe is brought in for intraoperative flow measurements.

9.8.12 Last Maneuvers

In arrested heart TECAB and after pump supported beating heart TECAB the patient is weaned from cardiopulmonary bypass and decannulated. A short phase of respiratory compromise, probably due to the combination of single-lung ventilation and cardiopulmonary bypass, needs to be expected. Usually this phase is self-limited. Once adequate pump function without signs of myocardial ischemia is ensured protamine is given. A tracheal suction tube is brought in through the parasternal assistance port and residual blood is evacuated from the pleural space. The thoracic cavity is thoroughly inspected for bleeding and cauterization maneuvers are carried out as needed. Once adequate hemostasis is confirmed the robotic system is undocked. It is important to leave all ports in place. They are removed under direct videoscopic vision and the portholes are cauterized from outside if necessary. A chest tube is inserted through the camera porthole. This maneuver should be done with the left lung inflated so as to avoid injuries to the graft during tube insertion. The portholes are then closed.

9.9 Postoperative Care

Postoperative treatment after robotic coronary artery bypass grafting follows the general principles applied in open CABG. Some specifics, however, need to be taken into consideration. There are currently no temporary pacing wires which can be placed endoscopically. For this reason patients go to the intensive care unit without external pacing wires and other methods of temporary pacing such as endovenous or transthoracic are used if necessary. Patients during TECAB have undergone double-lumen tube intubation and single-lung ventilation; therefore, respiratory compromise can occur and the postoperative chest x-ray may show increased rates of atelectasis as compared to open surgery through sternotomy. Occasionally the postoperative ventilation time is prolonged. Weaning from the ventilator follows general principles. Adequate postoperative respiratory therapy is important. Dyspnea will vanish with loss of extracellular fluid and generalized edema through diuresis.

Patients will arrive at the ICU with unilateral or bilateral pleural tubes placed through the camera porthole or through separate chest tube incisions. The camera porthole is relatively painful until the chest tube is removed and additional pain control may be necessary. One major advantage in TECAB is that the sternum is completely intact. Therefore mobilization throughout the whole postoperative course faster than in open CABG through sternotomy is facilitated. No sternal precautions are ordered.

In patients in whom a hybrid coronary revascularization concept is pursued, dual antiplatelet (DAP) therapy needs special attention. When surgery is done first the interval between TECAB and percutaneous coronary intervention (PCI) is bridged with DAP therapy so as to avoid interval plaque destabilization and myocardial ischemia. In patients who have received PCI before TECAB or in those who undergo simultaneous coronary intervention continuation of DAP therapy is of utmost importance.

In TECAB cases without intraoperative technical challenges bleeding rates are usually minimal. The chest tube container will be filled with a small amount of blood followed by a phase of relatively significant serosanguinous and serous drainage. Chest tube removal is possible realistically on postoperative day two or three with discharge from the hospital usually shortly thereafter. Our current data have shown that the main factors influencing hospital stay are the surgical learning curve, technical difficulties resulting in conversion to sternotomy, and revision for bleeding [4]. All these factors are likely to be controlled with growing experience of robotic surgery teams.

The main advantages of robotic endoscopic CABG are visible in the early rehabilitation phase [5]. Time to return to everyday activity is reduced. Sternal precautions after CABG through sternotomy limit the patient up to 12 weeks, whereas patients after TECAB can resume strenuous activities within 3–4 weeks. Driving can be allowed as soon as patients are off narcotic pain medications and if no obvious confusion is present. Patients can be allowed to lift weight, push, and pull as usually immediately after discharge.

9.10 General Role of the Procedure and Stepwise Implementation

TECAB is currently performed at very few centers worldwide and is one of the most complex procedures in surgery. Complexity translates into learning curves, increased operative times, and cost. According to the experience of the four teams we worked with, the benefits are very well worth the efforts, however. Patients appreciate the high-tech aspect of the procedure and most often decide for TECAB if they are offered the option. Patients find TECAB programs on the internet and travel to experienced centers. The feedback from patients who recover from CABG within 3–4 weeks is highly motivating.

Individual surgeons and hospitals offering a TECAB service appreciate the atmosphere of a modern surgical environment. From the ergonomic perspective robotic surgery is attractive because the surgeon works without headlights, loops, and gown. From the surgical infection point of view the procedure is also attractive. The thoracic interior is not as exposed to the outside environment and deep thoracic wound infections can potentially be reduced. The blood contact of the surgical team is also limited offering additional protection if patients with blood-derived infectious disease are treated.

It is very important to approach the initiation of a TECAB program in a stepwise manner. The whole team including cardiologists, surgeons, assistants, perfusionists, anesthesiologists, hospital administrators and postoperative caregivers should be involved and a detailed treatment protocol should be developed. The surgeons must practice robotic surgery in simulations using dry-lab and wet-lab models. We recommend at least 100 anastomoses sutured in cadaver pig hearts before suturing in the clinical setting. Both IMA harvesting and anastomotic suturing should first be performed in regular open CABG cases and not primarily in TECAB. Experience with remote access heart-lung machine perfusion and the use of the endoballoon must be gained in other minimally invasive procedures before using these delicate techniques in TECAB. If such a stepwise approach is taken, safe implementation of a challenging but highly attractive procedure can be expected.

References

1. Bonatti J, Schachner T, Bonaros N, Lehr E, Zimrin D, Griffith B (2011) Robotic assisted endoscopic coronary bypass surgery. Circulation 124:236–244
2. Bonatti J, Lehr E, Vesely M, Schachner T, Bonaros N, Zimrin D (2010) Hybrid coronary revascularization: which patients, when, how. Curr Opin Cardiol 25:568–574
3. Bonatti J, Wehman B, De Biasi AR, Griffith B, Lehr EJ (2012) Totally endoscopic quadruple coronary artery bypass grafting is feasible using robotic technology. Ann Thorac Surg 5:111–112
4. Lee JD, Bonaros N, Hong P, Srivastava M, Herr D, Lehr EJ, Bonatti J (2013) Factors influencing hospital length of stay after robotic totally endoscopic coronary artery bypass. Ann Thorac Surg 95:813–818
5. Bonaros N, Schachner T, Wiedemann D, Oehlinger A, Ruetzler E, Feuchtner G, Kolbitsch C, Velik-Salchner C, Friedrich G, Pachinger O, Laufer G, Bonatti J (2009) Quality of life improvement after robotically assisted coronary artery bypass grafting. Cardiology 114:59–66

Robotic Surgery for Mitral Valve Disease

Tsuyoshi Kaneko, Bryan Bush, Wiley Nifong, and W. Randolph Chitwood Jr.

10.1 Introduction

Mitral valve surgeries have been performed traditionally through a median sternotomy. However, over the past two decades, minimally invasive mitral valve surgery has evolved as important option for cardiac surgeons and patients. Improvements in instruments and endoscopes and patient demand have pushed this field farther. Cohn et al published a large series using a lower hemisternotomy with comparable outcomes to conventional surgery [1].

Video-assisted surgery started to take place after the accumulated experience with direct vision operations through right mini-thoracotomy and additional development of the endoscopic device. In 1996, Carpentier reported the first case of video-assisted mitral valve repair through right mini-thoracotomy [2].

With the recent progress in robotic technology, utilizing the da Vinci™, telemanipulation system model (Intuitive Surgical, Inc., Sunnyvale, CA, USA) now allows surgeons to perform keyhole surgery with full wrist-like articulations. This device was first utilized by Carpentier in 1998 to perform the first endoscopic mitral valve repair using an early prototype of the da Vinci™ [3]. The first robotic mitral valve repair in North America was performed by Chitwood in 2000 [4]. Subsequent Food and Drug Administration (FDA) approval of this system was obtained in 2002 for mitral valve surgery after successful phase I and II multicenter FDA trials. With advances in visualization, instrument ergonomics, and ease of use by the surgical

---

T. Kaneko, M.D.
Department of Cardiac Surgery, Brigham and Women's Hospital, Harvard Medical School, Boston, MA, USA

B. Bush, M.D. • W. Nifong, M.D. • W.R. Chitwood Jr., M.D., FACS, FRCS (✉)
Department of Cardiovascular Sciences, Brody School of Medicine, East Carolina Heart Institute, East Carolina University, Greenville, NC 27858, USA
e-mail: chitwoodw@ecu.edu

staff, robotic cardiac surgery is becoming more standardized and the application in cardiac surgery has been growing.

10.2 Indication and Exclusion Criteria

All degenerative, ischemic, and rheumatic mitral valve disease is considered for treatment by robotic mitral surgery. Patients with atrial fibrillation can be surgically treated simultaneously by a robotic CryoMaze (Cox IV) procedure. Tricuspid disease can be surgically managed through robotic approach as well.

Patients requiring aortic surgery, aortic valve surgery and/or coronary artery bypass are considered for conventional sternotomy approach. Previous contraindications for robotic mitral surgery have included a poor ejection left ventricular ejection fraction (<35 %), a previous cardiac operation, a right thoracotomy, or severe aortoiliac vascular disease. However, today we have expanded the indications. We perform axillary artery cannulation using an 8-mm sidearm PTFE graft in the presence of either small or atherosclerotic femoral vessel. This technique is used most often in elderly patients and for reoperations. Currently, we now use robotic techniques for reoperations in patients who have had a prior sternotomy.

Absolute exclusion criteria include patients with a severely calcified mitral valve annulus, a prior right-side lung resection, severe pulmonary hypertension (PAS > 70 mmHg), a very poor left ventricle (EF < 25 %), and/or right ventricular failure.

10.3 Preoperative Workup

The transthoracic echocardiogram (TTE) and/or transesophageal echocardiogram (TEE) are used to assess the exact etiology of the mitral valve disease. Cardiac catheterization is performed in patients over forty years old to rule out possible coronary disease. Carotid ultrasound is reserved for high-risk patients. Whole-body computed tomography and femoral arterial ultrasound are performed in on high-risk patients to predict the risk of femoral cannulation. Pulmonary function tests are performed on high-risk patients to assess the adequate pulmonary reserve needed for one-lung ventilation. If poor lung function is present, cardiopulmonary bypass is initiated early for intracardiac access.

10.4 Preoperative Anesthesia

A double-lumen endotracheal tube or bronchial blocker is used to obtain single lung ventilation. Prior to sterile preparation of the patient, a pulmonary artery catheter and a 15–17-Fr Bio-Medicus™ (Medtronic, Inc., Minneapolis, MN, USA) arterial cannula for superior vena cava drainage are placed by the anesthesiologist using the Seldinger technique.

A pre-incision TEE is performed to evaluate the annular size, leaflet coaptation, leaflet lengthes, and risk for systolic anterior motion (SAM). We currently use anterior leaflet length, annular diameter, and septal thickness to select the annuloplasty ring size. Post-repair SAM can develop in patients with excess posterior leaflet tissue (posterior height >1.5 cm), a long anterior leaflet (>34 mm), left ventricular outflow tract septal hypertrophy, and in the presence of an acute angle (<120°) between the aortic and mitral annulus valve planes.

10.5 Operative Technique

Patients are placed on a left semi-lateral decubitus position with 30-degree right side elevation. Both arms are tucked with careful attention made to expose the axilla to leave enough space at the patient's side aortic cross clamp. The sternotomy line is marked, and parallel midclavicular, anterior axillary, and midaxillary lines are also marked for external guidance.

A four-centimeter mini-thoracotomy incision is made medial to the anterior axillary line. The pectoralis muscle is spared, and the fourth intercostal space is entered after the right lung is deflated. An alexis wound protector™ (Applied medical, Rancho Santa Margarita, CA) is applied to retract any soft tissue and to facilitate exchange of instruments and the camera. A pledgeted braided suture is placed in the central tendon of the diaphragm and pulled through the inferior chest wall using "crochet hook" for retraction and exposure entire pericardial.

Simultaneously, the right femoral artery and vein are dissected through a 2-cm oblique groin incision. Attention is made to make to incision close to the inguinal ligament. Purse-string sutures are placed in both vessels. Full-dose heparin is given after the diaphragm suture is placed. Under TEE guidance, a 22-Fr femoral venous cannula (Estech, San Ramon, CA, USA) is positioned in the central right atrium using the modified Seldinger technique. Similarly, the femoral artery is cannulated with either a 17- or 19-Fr Bio-Medicus™ arterial cannula. Using suction venous drainage, patients are cooled to 28 °C systemically.

Robotic trocars then are placed (Fig. 10.1). The trocar for the left atrial retractor is placed medial to the working incision. Injury to the internal mammary artery is carefully avoided during this trocar placement. The trocar for the left instrument arm is placed in the 3rd intercostal space at the anterior axillary line. The trocar for the right arm is placed in the 5th intercostal space slightly medial to midaxillary line. It is important to keep an 8–10-cm distance between the left and right arm in order to avoid intraoperative conflicts. An incision for aortic cross clamp and left atrial vent is made at this time.

The robot is then docked at the patient, and the pericardium is opened robotically 2 cm anterior to the phrenic nerve. The pericardial incision is extended in a smile fashion, aiming toward the sternum when opened superiorly and inferiorly. The pericardial retraction sutures are placed near the superior vena cava reflection and the atrio-inferior vena cava junction. A total of three pericardial sutures are placed the posterior edge and one is placed along the anterior edge. Posterior pericardial

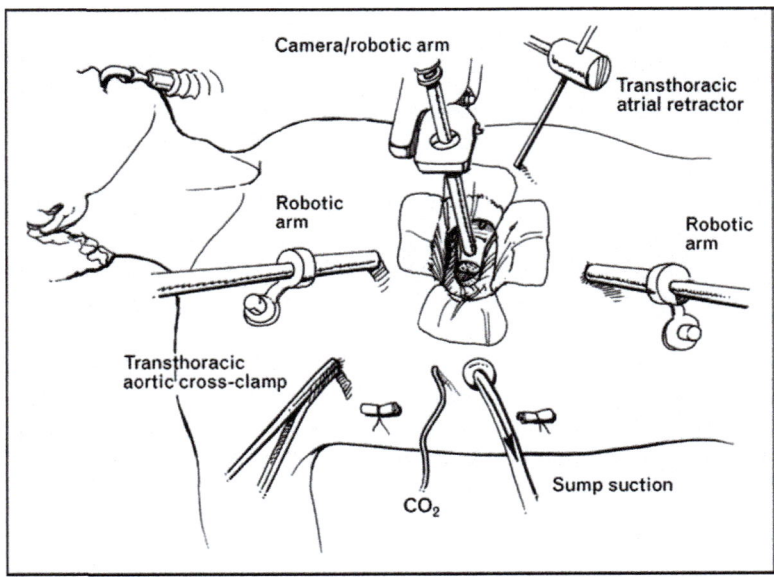

Fig. 10.1 Trocar position and setup for robotic mitral surgery. Reprinted from Anderson et al. [5] with permission from Wolters Kluwer health

retraction sutures are pulled posterior-laterally through the chest wall using a "crochet hook". A long cardioplegia needle is placed in the aortic root and a transthoracic aortic clamp (Scanlan, Inc., Minneapolis, MN, USA) is applied through the 2nd intercostal space just medial to anterior axillary line. To avoid conflicts with the left instrument arm, care is used to place the clamp as close to the axilla as possible. Direct visualization of the left atrium and pulmonary artery are important to avoid clamp injury. After the cross clamp is applied, the heart is arrested with antegrade cold cardioplegia.

After cardiac arrest, inter-atrial groove is dissected and the oblique sinus is opened behind the IVC. The left atriotomy is extended take out is made toward the oblique sinus. The robotic left atrial retractor is introduced, and ventral retraction is applied to elevate the interatrial septum for mitral valve exposure. A left atrial vent is placed in the left superior pulmonary vein.

10.6 Mitral Valve Repair/Replacement

10.6.1 Posterior Leaflet Prolapse

Posterior leaflet prolapse is the most common cause of myxomatous mitral valve regurgitation. Etiologies include redundant leaflets, ruptured chordae, elongated papillary muscles, and widened leaflet indentations. Robotic micro-scissors and atraumatic forceps are used for leaflet resections. Leaflet resections are performed by triangular, trapezoidal, or quadrangular resection of the prolapsed leaflet.

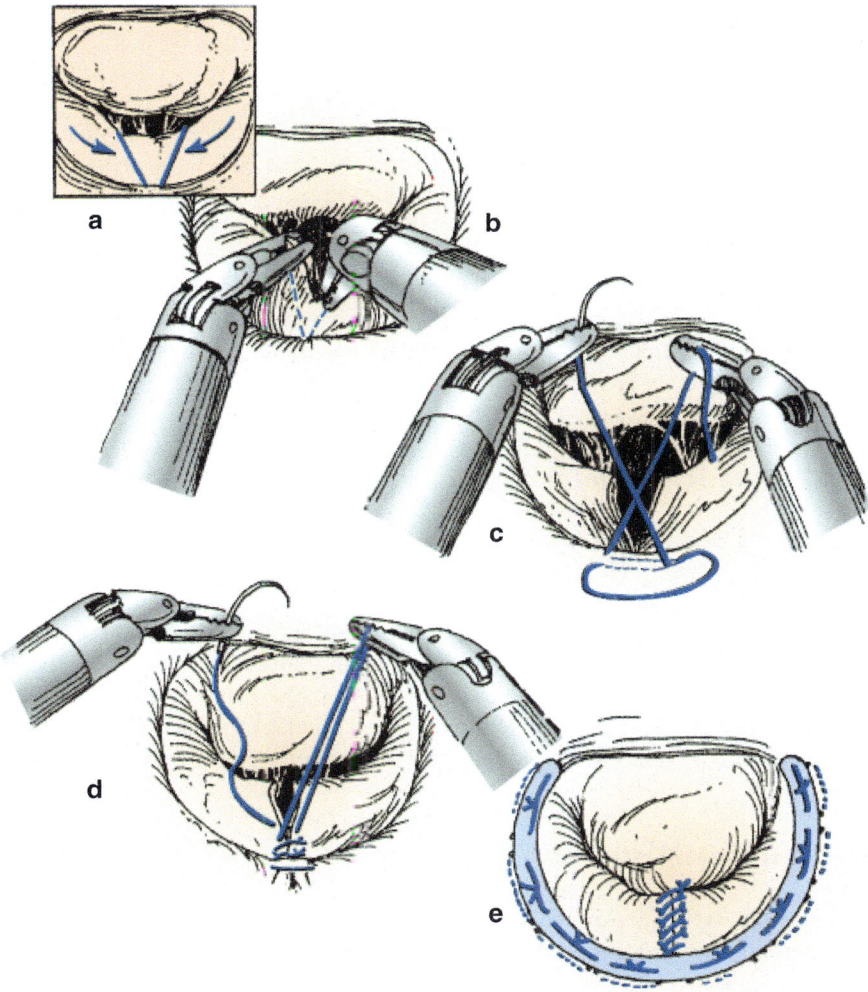

Fig. 10.2 Triangular resection of the posterior leaflet

Resections are performed to reduce posterior leaflets heights to at least 1.5 cm. It is important to identify nonfunctioning and functioning chordae and preserve the latter. Residual leaflet edges are approximated with 4-0 or 5-0 Cardionyl sutures (Peters Inc., Paris, France) (Fig. 10.2).

If SAM is a concern from a very long and redundant posterior leaflet, a sliding-plasty can be performed. This will move the anterior leaflet coaptation line away from the inter-ventricular septum and avoid SAM. Following a quadrangular resection of the prolapsed leaflet, leaflet remnant then is advanced along the annulus using a running suture. Both leaflet edges then are re-approximated as described above.

Another method to treat leaflet prolapse is by chordal replacement with a 5-0 or 4-0 PTFE suture (Gore-Tex™; Gore, Inc. Phoenix, AZ, USA). A short (16-cm) double-armed 4-0 Gore-Tex™ suture is passed in a figure-of-eight fashion through the papillary muscle fibrous head. Needles then are passed through the leaflet edge at the rupture/prolapse site and then around the coapting edge and back through the leaflet, creating a "locking loop." The second PTFE suture is placed in a similar fashion with a 3-mm gap between the sutures. Saline testing is done to assure correct neochordal length with optimal leaflet coaptation, and thereafter the sutures are tied down, avoiding knot slippage (Fig. 10.3).

10.6.2 Anterior Leaflet Prolapse

Currently, to treat anterior leaflet prolapse, we use chordal transfers and prosthetic chordal replacements. By swinging either basal (secondary) anterior leaflet or residual posterior leaflet primary chords to the anterior leaflet edge, this technique reduces the anterior leaflet prolapse. For significant anterior leaflet prolapse, multiple chords must be transferred. The defect in the posterior leaflet is repaired as described in the posterior leaflet prolapse section. Again the saline test is used to confirm the presence of residual regurgitation. Artificial chordal replacements are performed in the same fashion as described for posterior leaflet prolapse.

10.6.3 Annuloplasty/Valve Replacement

An annuloplasty is performed in conjunction with all leaflet repairs to reduce the annular size, prevent further dilatation, and restore the annular geometry. Also, by reducing the anterior-posterior diameter, a larger coaptation surface is created to prevent residual regurgitation. At our institution, flexible rings are used to treat myxomatous disease and complete rigid rings are used for ischemic disease.

For the flexible band, we use Cosgrove-Edwards™ (Edwards Lifesciences, Irvine, CA, USA) annuloplasty system. The band is removed from its holder for placement. Interrupted 2-0 braided sutures are used to attach the band, starting at the right fibrous trigone. To prevent kinking, the space between the two ring sutures should be narrow to secure sutures along the band. We use the Cor-Knot™ device (LSI Solutions, Inc., Victor, NY, USA). Interrupted horizontal mattress sutures are placed along the annulus in a clockwise fashion to the left fibrous trigone. Possible complications include injury to the circumflex artery near left posterior leaflet, aortic non-coronary cusp near left trigone, and conduction system near

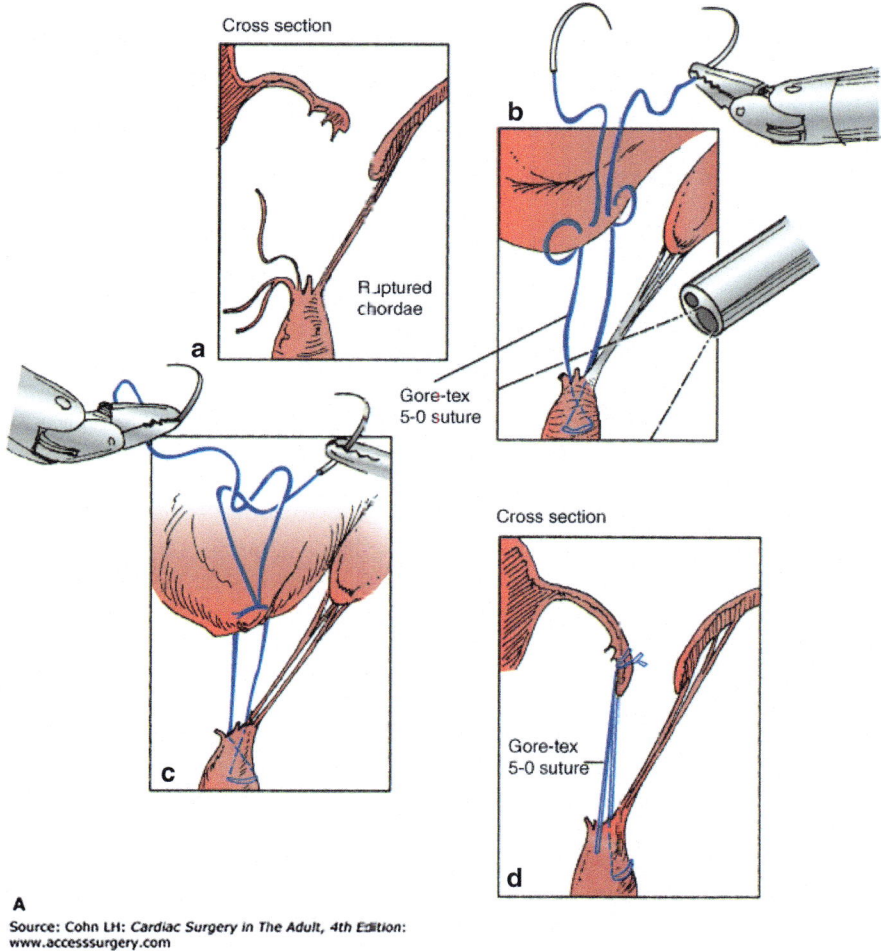

Fig. 10.3 Mitral valve repair using Gore-Tex neochordae

right trigone. This can be avoided by placing the needle perpendicular to the annulus without angling it. An alternative running suture method is used in some institutions [6].

Complete annuloplasty rings are placed using long braided double-arm sutures with suture holders placed around the working port. Horizontal mattress sutures are placed circumferentially. Then similar to open surgery, annular sutures are placed through the complete ring by the bed-side assistantextracorporeally. Then the ring is lowered to the annulus and secured with Cor-Knot™. Careful attention is made not to cross the sutures while placing them on the suture holder or annuloplasty ring. Robotic mitral valve replacements are performed similarly to complete ring annuloplasties. Both bioprosthetic and mechanical valve replacements are feasible with the robotic approach.

10.7 Current Experience

Over 800 robotic mitral valve operations have been performed using the da Vinci™ system at East Carolina University. Over 400 surgeons have been trained at our training program [7].

FDA approved this system for mitral valve surgery after successful phase I and II multicenter FDA trials in 2002. Since then, the da Vinci system has undergone three iterations of development, which has contributed to the expanded use of the device. The most recent da Vinci Si™ system has a fourth arm that can be used for left atrial dynamic retraction. This enables frequent changes in retraction to allow maximal exposure. With the recent advances in technology, more surgeons are adopting the robotic mitral approach into their practice.

Robotic access compared to other methods (full sternotomy, partial sternotomy, and mini-anterior-thoracotomy) had the lowest occurrence of atrial fibrillation and shortest hospitalization time by almost one day despite the longer operative, perfusion, and aortic cross-clamp times [8]. The robotic group also has better functional outcome including less pain and early return to work compared with traditional surgery [9].

Long operative, cardiopulmonary bypass and cross-clamp times may be shortened by using simplified mitral repair techniques, such as a running suture for the annuloplasty, triangular leaflet resections, folding plasties, artificial chordae for posterior leaflet [10], and the haircut posterior leaflet plasty [11]. Moreover, the use of the rapid suture attachment device, Cor-Knot™, has markedly decreased our annuloplasty prosthesis implantation time. Lastly, docking the robot instrument cart to the instrument trocars before beginning cardiopulmonary bypass aids in overall time economy during this operation.

The learning curve always plagues surgeons when they bring new, complex technology into clinical practice. The learning curve shoulder is considered to be approximately 50 robotic mitral valve repair cases [12]. Our current recommendation is for surgeons to become comfortable with right mini-thoracotomy mitral repairs before advancing to the robotic approach. This progression will advance teamwork and instill confidence in the surgeon, the operating room nurses, and the anesthesia team.

To date, we have completed over 800 robotic mitral valve surgeries with the da Vinci™ system and have published results on the first 540 [13]. There was a 0.4 % (2) thirty-day mortality and a 1.7 % (9) late mortality. This series did not include mitral valve replacements. Complications included three (0.6 %) strokes, one transient ischemic attack, four (0.7 %) myocardial infarctions, and thirteen (2.4 %) reoperations for bleeding. The mean hospital stay was 5.6 ± 4.0 days.

Sixteen (2.9 %) patients required a midterm or late reoperation. From these data we concluded that robotic mitral valve repair was safe and associated with good midterm durability.

10.8 Conclusion

Robotic cardiac surgery is still evolving despite being deployed for over a decade. Improved optics and instrumentation, progressively smaller incisions, simulated three-dimensional vision, and enhanced surgeon hand-eye coordination all will become a major part of our surgical future. Despite this optimistic view, many surgeons remain concerned with the complexity and procedure cost that they will not adopt this platform. However, it is clear that developing technology will further robotic surgery evolution and eventually provide more comfort for these surgeons. The learning curve still remains an issue; however, training systems may be able to model most surgical procedures through immersive technology in the future [14]. Nevertheless, robot-assisted mitral valve surgery has developed to become a safe and successful modality.

References

1. Cohn LH, Adams DH, Couper GS et al (1997) Minimally invasive cardiac valve surgery improves patient satisfaction while reducing costs of cardiac valve replacement and repair. Ann Surg 226:421–426
2. Carpentier A, Loulmet D, LeBret E et al (1996) Chirurgie a coeur ouvert par video-chirurgie et mini-thoracotomie- primier cas (valvuloplastie mitrale) opere avec succes [First open heart operation (mitral valvuloplasty) under videosurgery through a minithoracotomy]. Comptes Rendus De L'Academie des Sciences: Sciences de la vie 319:219–223
3. Carpentier A, Loulmet D, Aupecle B et al (1998) Computer assisted open-heart surgery. First case operated on with success. CR Acad Sci II 321:437–442
4. Chitwood WR Jr, Nifong LW, Elbeery JE et al (2000) Robotic mitral valve repair: trapezoidal resection and prosthetic annuloplasty with the da Vinci surgical system. J Thorac Cardiovasc Surg 120:1171–1172
5. Anderson CA, Kypson AP, Chitwood WR (2008) Robotic mitral surgery: current and future roles. Curr Opin Cardiol 23:117–120
6. Mihaljevic T, Jarrett CM, Gillinov AM et al (2010) A novel running annuloplasty suture technique for robotically assisted mitral valve repair. J Thorac Cardiovasc Surg 139(5):1343–1344
7. Kypson AP, Nifong LW, Chitwood WR Jr (2004) Robot-assisted surgery: training and re-training surgeons. Int J Med Robot Comput Assist Surg 1:70–76
8. Mihaljevic T, Jarrett CM, Gillinov AM et al (2011) Robotic repair of posterior mitral valve prolapse versus conventional approaches: Potential realized. J Thorac Cardiovasc Surg 141:72–80
9. Suri RM, Antiel RM, Burkhart HM et al (2012) Quality of life (QOL) after early mitral valve repair using conventional and robotic approaches. Ann Thorac Surg 93:761–769
10. Mihaljevic T, Pattakos G, Gillinov AM et al (2013) Robotic posterior mitral leaflet repair: neochordal versus resectional techniques. Ann Thorac Surg 95(3):787–794

11. Chu MW, Gersch KA, Rodriguez E et al (2008) Robotic "haircut" mitral valve repair: posterior leaflet-plasty. Ann Thorac Surg 85(4):1460–1462
12. Suri RM, Burkhart HM, Daly RC et al (2011) Robotic mitral valve repair for all prolapse subsets using techniques identical to open valvuloplasty: establishing the benchmark against which percutaneous interventions should be judged. J Thorac Cardiovasc Surg 142:970–979
13. Nifong LW, Rodriguez E, Chitwood WR (2012) 540 consecutive robotic mitral valve repairs including concomitant atrial fibrillation cryoablation. Ann Thorac Surg 94:38–43
14. Meir AH, Rawn CL, Krummel TM (2001) Virtual reality: surgical application-challenge for the new millennium. J Am Coll Surg 192:372–384

Robotic Surgery in General Thoracic Surgery

Hyun-Sung Lee and Hee-Jin Jang

11.1 Introduction

Minimally invasive surgery (MIS) has been an important treatment modality in many fields of surgery. However, in the field of MIS, the advance of thoracic surgery has been delayed due to limited thoracic space with fixed rib cages, a beating heart, and ventilation of the lungs. The ergonomic discomfort and counterintuitive instruments have hindered the application of video-assisted thoracic surgery (VATS) to more advanced procedures. Initially, VATS was used as a diagnostic tool. With the development of thoracoscopic instruments and vision systems, VATS has been applied to major thoracic surgery, such as a pulmonary lobectomy. Successful thoracoscopic surgery is highly surgeon-dependent and requires a high degree of dexterity and technical skill. The uncomfortable operative position and the flat, two-dimensional view made it one of the most difficult operations, requiring a long learning curve. Because MIS has been proven to be beneficial to the patients, broadening its use has become an important issue.

Trials to alleviate the shortcomings of VATS have developed the robotic technology. The use of robotic assistance during MIS was first described in 1985 [1], and the technology has evolved to its current state in the form of the *da Vinci* surgical system® (Intuitive Surgical, Sunnyvale, CA, USA) [2]. This technology offers several creative advantages, including a three-dimensional view of the operative field, absence of a fulcrum effect, seven degrees of freedom of movement

---

H.-S. Lee, M.D., Ph.D. (✉) • H.-J. Jang, M.D.
Department of Systems Biology, Division of Cancer Medicine,
University of Texas MD Anderson Cancer Center, 7435 Fannin Street,
2SCR3 3205, Houston, TX, USA 77054
e-mail: hyunsungleethoracic@gmail.com; hlee10@mdanderson.org;
catherine.of.siena429@gmail.com; hjang@mdanderson.org

with "wristed" instruments (*EndoWrist*®) that facilitate intracorporeal suturing, elimination of surgeon tremor, and ergonomic benefits. Thus, robotic assistance has consistently reproducible advantages over open approaches, including smaller incisions, reduced intraoperative blood loss, decreased postoperative pain, and shorter hospital lengths of stay (LOS) and convalescence periods. The disadvantages of robot-assisted surgery include the absence of tactile feedback and instrument collisions when traversing wide surgical fields [3–18].

Although the *da Vinci* system was originally intended for cardiac surgeries [19], it has found widespread applications across multiple specialties, with the vast majority of cases dedicated toward oncologic procedures. We present here our robotic surgery for lung cancer and mediastinal tumors using the *da Vinci* Surgical System® with literature reviews.

11.2 Robotic Surgery in Lung Cancer

The standard treatment for stage I non-small cell lung cancer (NSCLC) is a lobectomy with mediastinal lymph node dissection (MLND). This standard of care was effectively established by the landmark publication from the Lung Cancer Study Group in 1995 demonstrating decreased local recurrence rates and a trend toward improved survival after a lobectomy compared with sublobar resections, including anatomic segmentectomies requiring individual pulmonary arterial and bronchial division and nonanatomic pulmonary wedge resections [20]. In 2007, a prospective, multi-institutional study to examine the standardized, truly videoscopic, minimally invasive VATS lobectomy procedure for early-stage lung cancer showed that a VATS lobectomy is feasible. The low complication rates and short duration of chest tube placement suggest there may be a benefit to the patient; furthermore, at early follow-up, the secondary survival end point compared favorably with that in the open lobectomy series [21]. A VATS lobectomy has been reported to be beneficial for patients, with more favorable early postoperative outcomes and long-term oncologic outcomes that are comparable with an open lobectomy [22–28]. Despite these advantages, a recent analysis of the voluntary Society of Thoracic Surgery (STS) database demonstrated that although the percentage of all lobectomies performed by VATS has been increasing, the overall percentage of cases performed by VATS during the 3-year study period ending in 2006 was only 20 %, possibly due to the limitations of visualization and maneuverability of the approach [29]. However, the majority of major lung resections performed in the USA are still via thoracotomy.

Some pioneers have challenged to perform robot-assisted video-assisted thoracic surgery (R-VATS) pulmonary resection. Based on the literature review of R-VATS pulmonary resection (Table 11.1), the operative time was 3.3 h. Open conversions were required in 6 %, and the LOS was 5 days. Overall, complications occurred in less than 20 %. Death occurred in 1 %. Conversions, operative times, LOS, complications, mortality, and oncologic outcomes were consistent with previous

Table 11.1 Reviews of R-VATS pulmonary resections

Authors	Year	No.	Conversion	Op. time (h)	LOS (day)	Cx (%)	Mortality (%)
Melfi [16]	2005	23	2	3.2	5 (1.3)	NR	NR
Park [17]	2006	34	4	3.6 (2.6–5.9)	4.5 (2–14)	26	0
Anderson [3]	2007	31	0	3.6 (1.0–6.4)	4 (2–10)	27	0
Gharagozloo [11]	2008	100	0	4.0 (3.0–6.0)	4 (3–42)	21	3
Venonesi [18]	2010	54	7 (13 %)	3.9 (2.4–8.5)	4.5 (3–24)	20	0
Giulianotti [12]	2010	38	6 (15.8 %)	3.5 (1.8–6.3)	10 (3–24)	10.5	2.6
Cerfolio [8]	2011	106	11 (10.4 %)	2.2 ± 0.4	2 (1–7)	27	0
Dylewski [9][a]	2011	200	3 (1.5 %)	1.5 (0.5–4.65)	3 (1–44)	26	1.5
Jang [14][b]	2011	40	0	4.0 ± 0.0	6 (4–22)	10	0
Lee [31][b]	2012	100	2 (2 %)	3.5 ± 1.0	6.3 ± 3.3	9	0
Park [38][c]	2012	325	27 (8.3 %)	3.4 (1.8–6.4)	5 (2–28)	25	0.3
Overall		1,031	62 (6 %)	3.3	4.9	17.6	0.8

R-VATS = robot-assisted video-assisted thoracic surgery
[a]Benign diseases were included in this study
[b]Twenty patients overlapped in these studies
[c]This is a multicenter study from the USA and Italy

reports of VATS outcomes. The robotic approach confers advantages over open surgery similar to VATS [3–5, 7–9, 11, 12, 14, 17, 18, 30, 31]. However, as existing data do not demonstrate superiority over VATS, comparative effectiveness studies are needed to explore short-term outcomes, such as pain and respiratory function, and to assess cost differences.

11.2.1 Robot-Assisted VATS (R-VATS) Lobectomy for Lung Cancer

11.2.1.1 Indication

As in a VATS lobectomy, early-stage lung cancer is the indication for robotic surgery. The indication for robotic surgery can be modified according to different features, such as the tumor size, the extent of pleural adhesion, incomplete fissure, and the presence of calcified and anthracotic lymph nodes (LN).

11.2.1.2 Patient Position

During a thoracotomy, the patient is usually placed in a slightly flexed left lateral decubitus position to widen the intercostal space. During robotic surgery, the patient is more flexed to avoid the collision between the 30° thoracoscope and the pelvis and was then moved to a 10-degree reverse-Trendelenburg position. For a

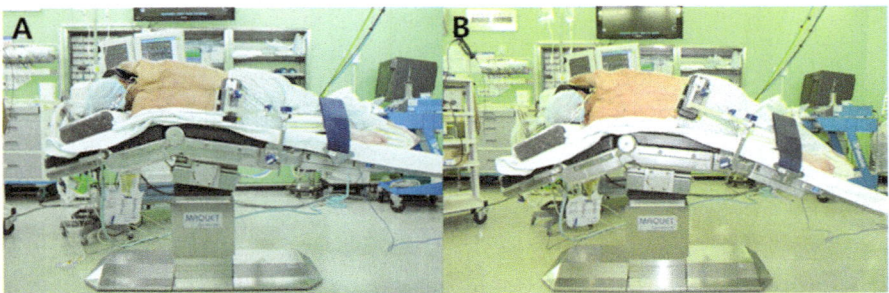

Fig. 11.1 Position of patients. (**a**) During thoracotomy or VATS. (**b**) During R-VATS

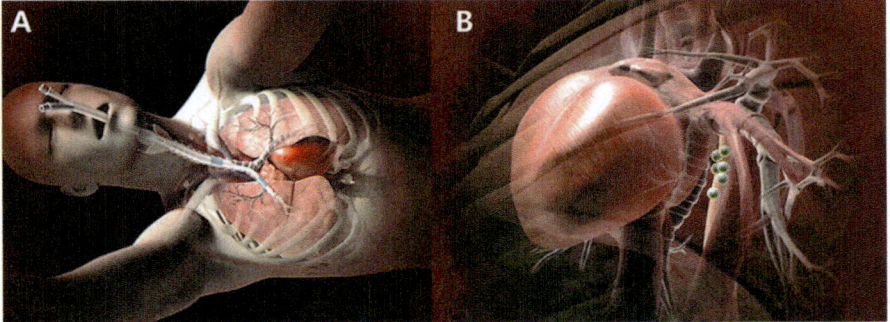

Fig. 11.2 Anterior approach to the subcarinal LNs with right-sided double-lumen endotracheal tube intubation during left sided R-VATS. (**a**) A right-sided double-lumen endotracheal tube is inserted into the right bronchus. (**b**) During R-VATS, subcarinal LNs can be dissected anteriorly

woman with a large pelvis, a 30-degree thoracoscope might be changed to 0° to prevent damage to her pelvis (Fig. 11.1).

The robotic cart approach to the patient in an oblique manner is helpful to reach the inferior pulmonary ligament and to permit enough space for the assistant standing on the anterior side of the patient.

11.2.1.3 Anesthesia

During right-sided R-VATS lobectomy, a double-lumen endotracheal tube was inserted into the left main bronchus. In contrast, during left-sided R-VATS lobectomy, a right-sided double-lumen endotracheal tube was inserted into the right bronchus (Fig. 11.2). This approach enabled the left main bronchus to be easily lifted during subcarinal LN dissection. For full anesthesia, fentanyl and vecuronium were infused continuously.

11.2.1.4 Selection of Robotic Instruments

Despite many diverse instruments, the cost of instruments is very expensive, and the number of uses is limited; thus, the selection should be deeply considered. Also, the insurance reimbursement system can affect the selection of the instruments.

We selected fenestrated bipolar forceps to grasp the lung parenchyma to prevent the injury. Additionally, these forceps are safe to grasp pulmonary veins. A bipolar energy source is added to control the bleeding from small vessels and lymphatics. *Cadiere*® forceps and ProGrasp® forceps have the same shape. However, *Cadiere*® forceps have no energy source, and ProGrasp® forceps have grasping power strong enough to injure the lung parenchyma and vessels.

Robotic ultrasonic devices can be used during robotic surgery. However, the cost is more expensive, and the motion of ultrasonic devices is limited due to the absence of wrist motion. We believe that a bipolar energy source and endostaplers are enough to complete the pulmonary lobectomy. Robotic instruments have continued to evolve, and robotic stapling devices will be launched in the future. However, the cost-effectiveness should be considered.

11.2.1.5 Robot-Assisted Pulmonary Resection with Four Arms

In the case of the right approach, a "utility incision" is made with 3–5 cm length at the fifth ICS along the anterior axillary line through the submammarian line, where the right robotic arm ① is placed. The camera port is placed at the seventh ICS along the mid-axillary line for the 30-degree 3D scope, and the other port is placed at the seventh ICS along the post-axillary line for the left robotic arm ②. An additional 5-mm port is placed at the seventh ICS around the auscultatory triangle at the back side for the robotic arm ③ (Fig. 11.3). Port placement between the right and left sides is consistent regardless of tumor location and tumor site. Occasionally, the submammarian incision in women is located at the sixth ICS. In that case, the other ports should move to the eighth ICS.

Wound protractors (Alexis®, Applied Medical, Rancho Santa Margarita, CA, USA) are inserted into three incision sites except 5-mm port to prevent tumor contamination and port-site bleeding from muscle tears. In addition, the application of wound protractors reduces the docking time because the robotic arm is directly inserted with the robotic trocar already docked.

For the robotic arm ① and ②, bipolar fenestrated forceps and the spatula-type monopolar electrocautery *EndoWrist*® are used. The dissection and anatomical isolation of the hilar structures are performed using two arms of the *da Vinci* system®. For the robotic arm ③, the thoracic grasper is used. This instrument is commonly used when the lung parenchyma is retracted, and the mediastinal pleura is pulled during the LN dissection to provide a better surgical field. The docking of three cannulae and the camera port are performed. The dissection and anatomical isolation of the hilar structures are performed using two arms of the *da Vinci* system®. The vessels and bronchus are usually ligated with thoracoscopic endostaplers (Multifire Endo GIA, Covidien, Mansfield, MA, USA). In some cases, the vessels are ligated with ties.

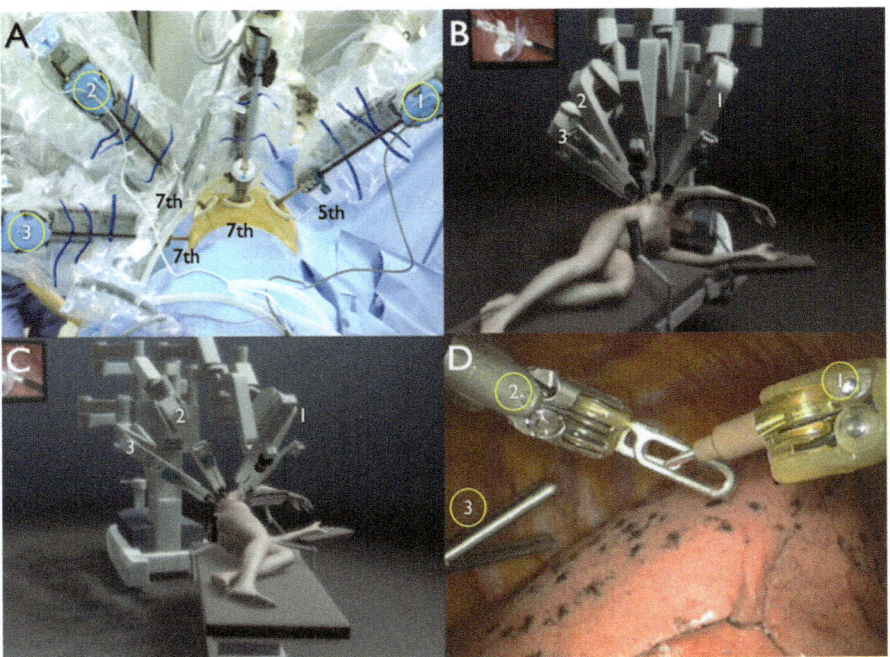

Fig. 11.3 Port placement and the use of instruments during robot-assisted pulmonary resection with four arms. (**a**) Port placement. (**b**) Cart approach (*anterior view*). (**c**) Cart approach (*foot view*). (**d**) Three instruments in the thoracic cavity (Reprinted from [31] with permission from Elsevier)

During upper lobectomies, the endostaplers are inserted through the posterior ports after the removal of the robotic arm. During lower lobectomies, the endostaplers are inserted through the utility port instead of removing the posterior robotic arm. The robotic arm through the utility incision can be removed out to achieve the wide angulation of endostaplers.

Our standard protocol involves complete LN dissection. After cessation of the procedure, an intercostal nerve block is routinely achieved with ropivacaine. After removal of the wound protractor, port-site bleeding is checked. A 24 Fr thoracic catheter is inserted through the camera port.

11.2.1.6 Mediastinal Lymph Node Dissection

Mediastinal LN staging is an important component of the assessment and management of patients with operable NSCLC and is necessary to achieve complete resection. One lingering criticism of the MIS approach is that LN dissection is inadequate compared with the thoracotomy approach. MLND is associated with more accurate staging, but whether MLND is associated with improved survival is not clear [32–37]. However, if the MIS technique is a viable treatment option for early-stage lung cancer, the performance of an equivalent oncologic resection, including adequate LN dissection similar in extent to open thoracotomy, is absolutely necessary.

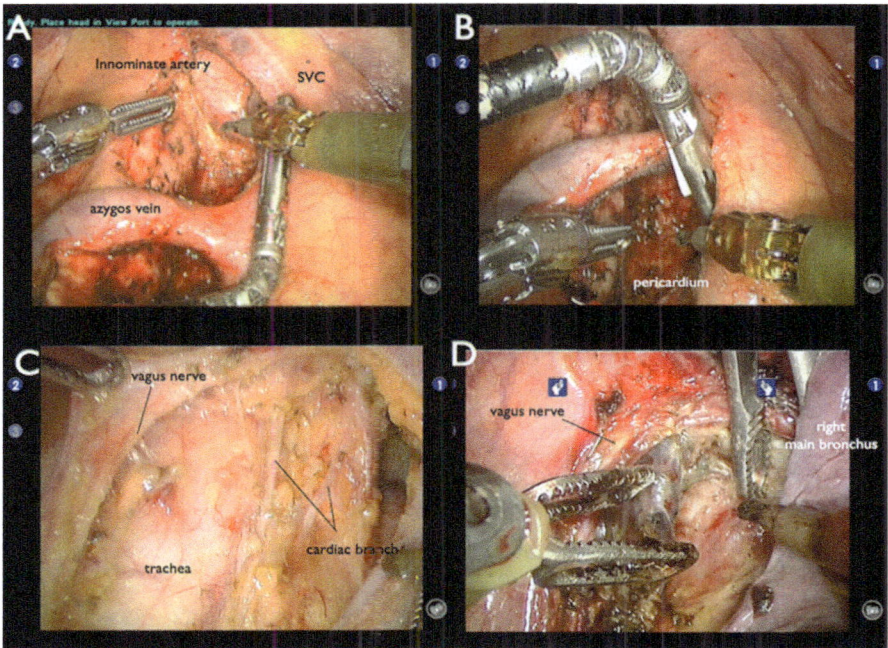

Fig. 11.4 Mediastinal lymph node dissection during a right-sided R-VATS lobectomy. (**a**) 2R. (**b**) 4R. (**c**) Cardiac branch from the vagus nerve in paratracheal space. (**d**) 7 (Reprinted from [31] with permission from Elsevier)

Right Paratracheal LNs (2R and 4R)

During paratracheal lymph node dissection (LND), the robotic arm ③ is very useful for retracting the superior vena cava (SVC) and the azygos vein. The mediastinal pleura, cephalad to the azygos vein (between the trachea and the SVC), is grasped with thoracic graspers and incised to the level of the innominate artery (Fig. 11.4a). A small vein draining from the mediastinal fat pad directly into the SVC is ligated with bipolar electrocautery.

The mediastinal fat pad is removed from the SVC to the trachea and from the cephalad border of the azygos vein to the caudal border of the innominate artery. A thoracic grasper in the robotic arm ③ is used to elevate the azygos vein, and the LNs that are located between its cephalic border and the origin of the bronchus of the right upper lobe are removed (Fig. 11.4b). During dissection at these levels, the lymphadenectomy may be extended to the contralateral LN levels (left paratracheal LN). Care must be taken not to injure the left recurrent laryngeal nerve, which is found in the tracheoesophageal groove. The cardiac branch from the vagus nerve before the trachea is the landmark of left deep border for right paratracheal LND (Fig. 11.4c).

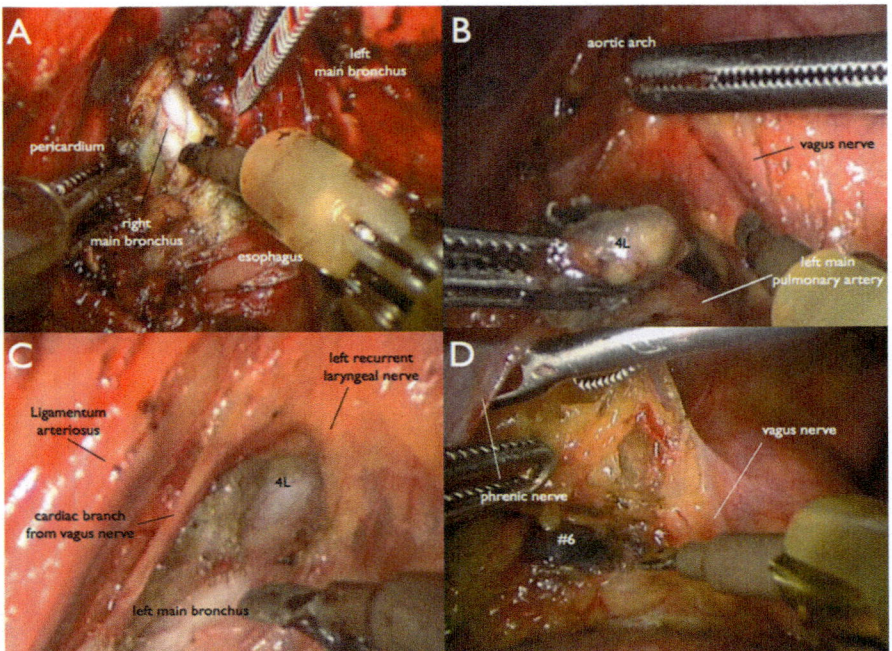

Fig. 11.5 Mediastinal lymph node dissection during a left-sided R-VATS lobectomy. (**a**) 7. (**b**) 4 L (during the removal). (**c**) 4 L (after removal). (**d**) 6 (Reprinted from [31] with permission from Elsevier)

Subcarinal LNs (During Right R-VATS)

The attachments to the right and left main stems of the bronchi are performed with the right main bronchus up and the anterior side lifted using the robotic arm ③ (Fig. 11.4d). The subcarinal LN packet is grasped with bipolar fenestrated forceps. Before transection, vessels course along the anterior border of the trachea and enter the subcarinal LNs from the region of the carina. These arteries and veins must be identified and controlled with bipolar cautery before transection.

Subcarinal LNs During Left R-VATS

The *level 7* subcarinal LNs are approached with the lung retracted posteriorly during robotic surgery. The left main stem bronchus is identified and lifted up and posteriorly with the robotic arm ③. The LNs are grasped with bipolar fenestrated forceps, and the attachments to the left main bronchi are performed. At that time, the first assistant uses only one instrument—a long, curved, thin Yankauer sucker—to press the heart. The arterial vessel that commonly enters the LNs from the anterior border of the trachea at the level of the carina must be identified and ligated with bipolar cautery to avoid postoperative hemorrhage (Fig. 11.5a).

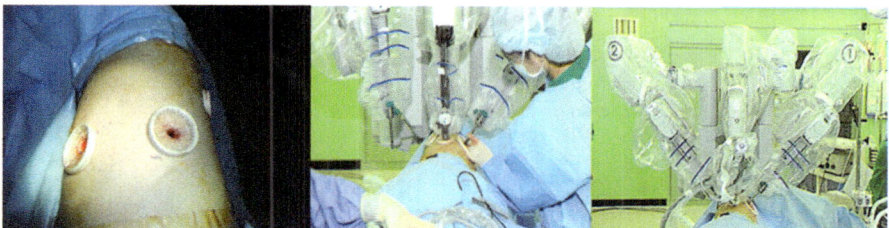

Fig. 11.6 Port placement of R-VATS with three arms

Left Paratracheal LNs (4 L)
The mediastinal pleura and the vagus nerve are lifted up with the robotic arm ③. The first assistant presses the left main pulmonary artery with the suction tip. The 4L LN is excised along the left main bronchus to the trachea with bimanual dissection (Fig. 11.5b, c). Because of the three-dimensional imaging and articulated arms, robotic surgery is very helpful for identifying the recurrent laryngeal nerve so that it is not injured.

Subaortic and Paraaortic LNs (5 and 6)
During the aortopulmonary window dissection, the mediastinal pleura with the phrenic nerve is tented with the robotic arm ③ (Fig. 11.5d).

11.2.1.7 Robot-Assisted Pulmonary Resection with Three Arms
All procedures are the same as the robot-assisted pulmonary resection with four arms except no additional 5 mm instrument is used (Fig. 11.6). Robot-assisted pulmonary resection with three arms depends more on the first assistant than that with four arms.

R-VATS with four arms and with three arms is compared in Table 11.2.

11.2.2 Robot-Assisted VATS (R-VATS) Segmentectomy

A pulmonary segmentectomy can be performed more delicately with robotic systems. Magnification and the articulated wrist are very helpful to approach the distal vascular and bronchial branches.

To determine the segment territory, air insufflation with a butterfly needle is used. Some reports have described air embolisms after air insufflation, but the magnified view can reduce the risk of an air embolism.

11.2.3 R-VATS Bronchoplasty or Sleeve Lobectomy

Intracorporeal suturing during MIS is a merit of robotic surgery. A bronchoplasty or sleeve lobectomy can be performed. In addition, angioplasty can be performed with bull dog clamping of the proximal and distal portion of the vessels. A bronchus

Table 11.2 Comparison between three-arm and four-arm robotic thoracic surgeries

View	Three-arm robotic surgery	Four-arm robotic surgery
Surgeon	– Easy to perform during the initial learning curve – Similar to VATS ports – More dependent on the assistant – Occasionally needs two assistants	– Needs more spatial sense – Less dependent on the assistant – Self-control of tissue retraction by the surgeon – During stapling, can use two robotic instruments
Assistant	– Two instruments in the narrow space – Robotic arm contamination – Injury to the assistant by the robotic arms – Collision between the robotic arms and VATS instrument – Uncomfortable insertion of endostaplers	– Increase in the resting time – Ability to focus on the surgical procedure – Better ergonomics – No physical injury – Reductions in collisions
Patient	– Same or similar number of incisions as VATS – Confined to two intercostal spaces	– Needs one more 5-mm incision and instrument – Meticulous dissection with the stable retraction of adjacent tissue according to the desires of the surgeon – Rare possibility of conversion
Nurse	– Prepares more VATS instruments	– Limited use of VATS instruments – Increased resting time by sitting

anastomosis has more tension, compared with the anastomosis of the intestines. Usually absorbable monofilament suture material is used for bronchial suturing during an open thoracotomy. During MIS, the knot of a monofilament suture can be loosened with ease. We use an interrupted suture with absorbable multifilaments to prevent the loosening of the knot. The robotic arm ③ is very useful for maintaining the tension of the bronchus by pulling up the suturing materials.

11.2.4 Technical Tips

11.2.4.1 Bleeding Control

Most surgeons are afraid of major bleeding during robotic surgery because the surgeon does not stand by the patient. Prevention is a high priority. During the robotic surgery, patience and anatomic knowledge are very important to prevent bleeding.

Once bleeding occurs, calmness without hesitation is very important, followed by compression of the bleeding site with robotic arms using gauze. This status can be maintained without difficulty with the robotic systems. Most bleeding can be controlled without conversion. A sealant such as Tachocomb® is also very useful to control bleeding. Additionally, a suture with prolene after clamping the vessels can be performed with a robotic system.

11.2.4.2 Pleural Adhesion

If there are some spaces to insert the robotic arms, pleural adhesion could be fully detached. During adhesiolysis, a 30-degree upward 3D thoracoscopic view is chosen. After detachment around the port sites, the thoracoscope can be changed to a 30-degree downward view.

Even if ventilation of one lung is unstable, robotic surgery could still proceed to completion within the small space. Thus, in the pediatric field, a robotic system can be applied to remove a mediastinal tumor.

11.2.4.3 Is CO_2 Insufflation During R-VATS Lobectomy Essential?

CO_2 insufflation can make the surgical field cleaner without smoke and bleeding. However, during robotic thoracic surgery, the surgical target is focused with magnification and can be approached more deeply and closely, depending on the control of the surgeon. Additionally, after the en bloc excision of the LN, the size of the excised LN is greater than 2 cm. These LNs would be squeezed during the removal through the 1.5-cm thoracoport, which is not oncologically safe. During the insertion and removal of the staplers, the leakage of CO_2 might be inconvenient. Additionally, a high intrathoracic pressure with CO_2 can cause hemodynamic deterioration. Attention should be paid to the potential of gas embolisms through the vascular stump site. During robot-assisted pulmonary resection for lung cancer, the merit of CO_2 seems to be very limited.

11.2.5 Learning Curves During Robotic Surgery in Lung Cancer

Some authors emphasized the faster learning curve of robotic surgery compared with that of VATS. The cutoff point was 20 cases [18]. However, from our experience, we needed approximately 50 cases to be confident regarding the use of robotic surgery for lung cancer due to the technical achievement of the anatomical complexity of the lungs. Based on our series, the operation time and console time were reduced after 30 cases (Fig. 11.7).

11.2.6 Long-Term Survival After R-VATS for Lung Cancer

Recently, long-term survival after robotic surgery for lung cancer has been reported from the USA and Italy [38, 39]. In 325 patients from three institutes, 310 patients were clinical stage I. The median follow-up was 27 months. The overall 5-year survival was 90 % in pIA, 88 % in pIB, 49 % in pII, and 43 % in pIII. Based on the 190 consecutive patients in our institute with a median follow-up of 26 months, the overall survival and disease-free survival for clinical stage I and II lung cancers were 91.4 % and 80 %, respectively. The overall 3 year survival was 98.1 % in pIA, 96.4 % in pIB, 96.2 % in pIIA, 80 % in pIIB, and 59.7 % in pIIIA (Fig. 11.8).

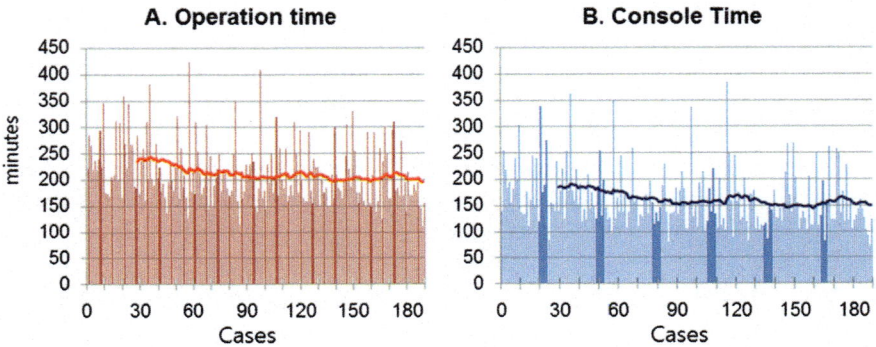

Fig. 11.7 Changes in the operation time (**a**) and console time (**b**) of R-VATS lobectomy for lung cancer

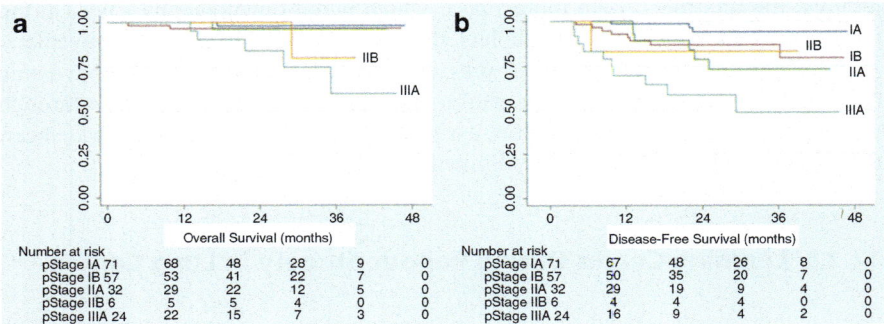

Fig. 11.8 Overall survival (**a**) and disease-free survival (**b**) after R-VATS lobectomy for lung cancer

The overall and stage-specific survivals are consistent with both the largest series of VATS lobectomies and the most recent data used for the revisions to the lung cancer staging system [40].

11.2.7 Comparison Between VATS and R-VATS Lobectomies for Lung Cancer

Two hundred consecutive lung cancer patients who underwent VATS or R-VATS lobectomies for clinical stage I and II NSCLCs were selected for comparison of the VATS and R-VATS lobectomy techniques [14, 31]. R-VATS lobectomies required longer surgical times than VATS lobectomies. However, the console time during the operation was similar to the operation time in the VATS lobectomies. The median length of the postoperative stay was significantly shorter after robotic surgery than after VATS (Table 11.3). Additionally, robotic surgery had a

Table 11.3 Postoperative results between R-VATS and VATS lobectomies for early-stage lung cancer

	R-VATS	VATS	p-value
Operation time (min)	209 ± 58	157 ± 40	<0.001
Console time (min)	155 ± 49	–	0.791
Dissected LN numbers	24.8 ± 8.8	23.6 ± 9.2	0.340
Nodal stations	7.3 ± 1.5	6.0 ± 1.4	<0.001
Time until discharge (days)	6.3 ± 3.3	8.9 ± 5.8	<0.001

Values are mean ± standard deviation. Reprinted from [31] with permission from Elsevier

Table 11.4 Postoperative complications between R-VATS and VATS lobectomies for lung cancer

	R-VATS (n = 100)	VATS (n = 100)	p-value
Conversion to thoracotomy	2	8	0.101
Postoperative mortality	0	2	0.497
Postoperative morbidity	9	21	0.028
Chylothorax	0	4	
Atrial fibrillation	2	1	
ALI or ARDS	1	3	
Prolonged air leak	4	10	
Sinus tachycardia	4	1	
Pulmonary artery thrombi	4	0	
Stump dehiscence	0	1	
Pericardial effusion	0	1	

ALI acute lung injury, *ARDS* acute respiratory distress syndrome

Table 11.5 Comparison of lymph node dissections between the VATS and R-VATS lobectomies

	VATS right	VATS left	R-VATS right	R-VATS left
Patients (n)	60	40	58	42
N2 MLN stations (n)	4.9 ± 1.0	4.7 ± 0.6	5.7 ± 1.2	5.3 ± 0.6
Individual LNs (n)	24.2 ± 9.8	22.7 ± 8.4	26.2 ± 9.3	22.9 ± 7.9

Reprinted from [31] with permission from Elsevier

significantly lower rate of postoperative complications. In the R-VATS lobectomies, two patients required a conversion to thoracotomy for oncologic reasons. However, in the VATS lobectomies, eight patients required a conversion to thoracotomy for mechanical, technical, and oncologic reasons (Table 11.4). The number of mediastinal LNs exceeded 20 for both the VATS and R-VATS procedures. The number of mediastinal nodal stations was approximately 5 in both procedures (Table 11.5).

11.2.8 Additional Comments

The key steps for performing an R-VATS pulmonary resection and MLND for early-stage lung cancer are as follows: (1) bimanual dissection, (2) dynamic exposure and adequate retraction with the robotic arm ③, (3) meticulous hemostasis, and (4) slow and steady techniques with perseverance.

A merit of robotic surgery is that bimanual dissection can be performed while the surgeon has autonomous control of both the camera and the instruments. To grasp the lung parenchyma and the node without damaging them, *Cadiere* forceps or fenestrated bipolar forceps are recommended. The grasping power is controllable by the surgeon once he has gained experience with the robot.

The dynamic exposure and retraction of tissues by utilizing all of the *da Vinci* instrument arms are essential to perform the en bloc resection of the mediastinal LNs. For right paratracheal LN dissection, the robotic arm ③ is helpful for pulling the SVC. Additionally, a minimal amount of help from an assistant is required for the retraction of the SVC and the azygos vein with the robotic arm ③.

For subcarinal LN dissection in the case of cancer of the right lung, the robotic arm ③ plays a role in lifting the main bronchus up, providing better exposure. The surgical field can be deepened to enable a closer approach, depending on the control of the surgeon.

Another advantage of the robotic system is the magnification. However, small bleeds can be magnified, and the surgical field may appear bloodier. Scrubbing LNs with a suction tip is not recommended because the surgical field becomes bloody. To maintain a clean view, meticulous hemostasis is essential. During robotic surgery, we usually use a monopolar cautery in the right hand and a bipolar cautery in the left hand. Secure control of the vessels and lymphatics is likely associated with decreased postoperative morbidities.

To complete an R-VATS pulmonary resection, the surgeon must have perseverance, which is more necessary during robotic surgery than during VATS or open thoracotomy. A common cause of conversion to thoracotomy during VATS is the presence of benign anthracotic and calcified LNs around the major vessels. However, a surgeon's slow and steady with an advanced robot-assisted system could provide an opportunity for a patient with severe anthracotic hilar LNs to undergo MIS without a conversion to open thoracotomy.

11.3 Robotic Surgery for Mediastinal Tumor

Given the early experiences of robotic surgery, the excision of a mediastinal tumor, such as a pericardial cyst or neurogenic tumor, can be performed. During the excision of mediastinal tumor, CO_2 insufflation is essential to widen the mediastinum and maintain the bloodless clean view. Because there is no need to use the endostaplers, the surgery can be performed by the surgeon alone. A first assistant is needed when the specimen is retrieved.

11.3.1 Anterior Mediastinal Tumor

In a patient with a thymoma, a total thymectomy by a median sternotomy has been universally accepted as the standard treatment. The VATS approach for a thymoma remains controversial, and many surgeons are reluctant to use this technique because of the supposed increased risk of local recurrence, reduced safety margins after minimally invasive resection, possible rupture of the capsule, and seeding of the tumor during endoscopic manipulations.

11.3.1.1 Robot-Assisted Thoracoscopic Thymectomy (R-VATS Thymectomy)

All surgeons have a policy of a "no-touch technique" with an en bloc resection of the thymus and perithymic fat tissue. During this technique, the thymoma is never touched, and normal thymic tissue and perithymic fat are used for grasping and for traction to avoid the direct manipulation of the tumor, capsular damage, and potential seeding. All thymic and perithymic fats are dissected with safe surgical margins, according to the International Thymic Malignancy Interest Group criteria [41], and the completeness of the thymectomy is assessed by the macroscopic inspection of both the thymic bed and the specimen [42].

The upper mediastinum is a delicate and difficult-to-reach anatomic area for a thoracoscopy, with large, vulnerable vessels and nerves. The two-dimensional view of the operative field, enhancement of the surgeon's tremor by the thoracoscopic instruments, and the inability of the instruments to articulate make it difficult to operate in a fixed, tiny three-dimensional space such as the mediastinum. Moreover, a thoracoscopic thymectomy is considered a technically challenging operation that requires a long learning curve [43]. The introduction of robotic surgical systems has added a new dimension to conventional thoracoscopy, providing additional advantages and overcoming some technical and methodological limits [42].

The main oncologic concerns are related to the possible breach of the tumor capsule, with the risk of tumor seeding locally or in the pleural cavity, and the difficult evaluation of the resection margins with reduced oncologic accuracy and safety. In our opinion, the robotic approach has some clear advantages compared with a conventional thoracoscopy. In fact, a lesser manipulation of the thymic and perithymic tissues is required during the operation, and a better evaluation of the healthy tissue as a result of the high-quality images leads to a more precise, lower risk dissection with wide safety margins and the reduced possibility of tumor breaching, incomplete resection, or iatrogenic injury. The use of carbon dioxide inflation (usually 8–12 mmHg) during the operation is another advantage, which allows enlargement of the mediastinal space with better visualization. The lack of tactile feedback could, theoretically, increase the risk of damaging the tumor tissue; however, this disadvantage appears to be compensated for by the superior three-dimensional visual control of the system.

We will now introduce Dr. Rückert's approach [42] and our preference for an R-VATS thymectomy. The approaches of R-VATS thymectomy through the right or left can be chosen based on the surgeon's preference:

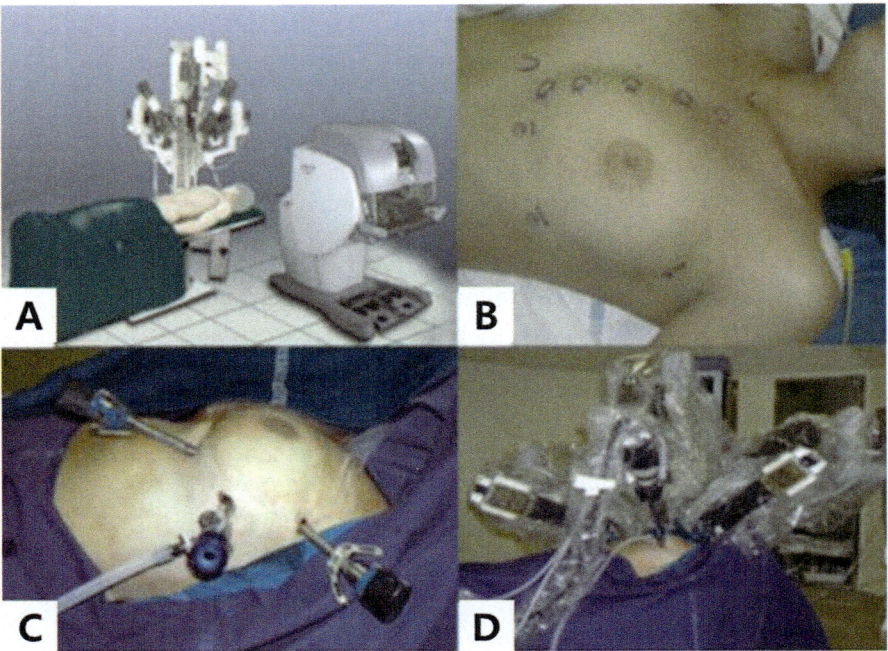

Fig. 11.9 Port placement and patient position during an R-VATS thymectomy (*left approach*). (**a**) In the surgical room, the patient is positioned supine on the surgical table with the left side elevated at 30°. The left arm is flexed on a support to expose the axillary region. The *da Vinci* robotic system with the surgical cart and the surgeon's console is displayed. (**b**) Before surgery, the fifth and third intercostal spaces (incision sites for port placement) are identified. The thoracic ports are placed, (**c**) and the arms of the robot are then attached to the ports and are operative. (**d**) Conflict between the arms should be avoided (Reprinted from [42] with permission from Elsevier)

1. **R-VATS thymectomy with a preference for the left approach by Dr. Rückert [42].**
   Dr. Ruckert and colleagues prefer the left approach in the left side upward position at a 30° angle using a bean bag. He uses the 0° 3D thoracoscope introduced through a 15-mm incision in the fifth ICS on the mid-axillary line. Care is taken when operating on the left side to avoid the heart, which lies just beneath this area. Thus, under camera vision and CO_2 insufflation to turn away the heart, two additional thoracic ports are inserted: one in the third ICS on the mid-axillary line and another in the fifth ICS between the parasternal and mid-clavicular lines. In women, three ports are lined along the submammarian line and its imaginary extension line to the axilla (Fig. 11.9).

   They prefer a left-sided approach for technical, clinical, and anatomical reasons. First, the left lobe of the thymus gland is usually larger and extends down to the pericardiophrenic area. The aortopulmonary window and the region below the left innominate vein are frequent sites of ectopic thymic tissue. In addition, by using the left-sided approach, they can easily demonstrate the right phrenic nerve to control complete resection [42].

The right-sided approach is reserved mainly for tumors located on the right side.

2. **R-VATS thymectomy with a preference for the right-sided approach.**
Despite the several merits of the left approach used by Dr. Rückert, routine left approaches may be avoided due to the fear of heart injury by the trocars and robotic instruments. The approach is instead decided by the tumor location. If the tumor deviates to the right, the right approach is selected; if the tumor deviates to the left, the left approach is selected. If the tumor is located at the midline, the right approach is selected because the right thoracic cavity is larger with minimal chance to injure the heart. In addition, the pericardium might be simultaneously resected for the en bloc resection of the tumor. However, a one-sided approach is insufficient to perform LN dissection and remove the cardiophrenic fat pad on the contralateral diaphragm. Frankly speaking, a one-sided approach can remove approximately two-thirds of the contralateral pericardial fat tissue. Therefore, for a total thymectomy, we prefer a bilateral approach using hybrid techniques (VATS and R-VATS).

First, in the contralateral side without the tumor, a 5-mm thoracoscope is used with two 5-mm thoracoscopic instruments under CO_2 insufflation (VATS phase). In the supine position with the left side slightly raised, cardiophrenic pericardial fat pad dissection is performed, and the phrenic nerve is identified and marked with clipping around the nerve, which is necessary to examine the margin of dissection from the contralateral approach. The 5-mm ultrasonic device is useful. During VATS, the upper part dissection can be skipped because the dissection of both upper parts of the thymus can be easily performed with R-VATS. During the dissection of the upper part of the thymus, the contralateral phrenic nerve can be identified. On the left side, the paraaortic and subaortic LNs are detached from the pericardium and the phrenic nerve; however, these are extracted during R-VATS from the right side. Three 5-mm stab wounds remain without chest tube insertion.

For R-VATS thymectomy (R-VATS phase), a patient is turned to the lateral decubitus position. The port placement is the same as that in an R-VATS lobectomy. A robotic thymectomy with four arms is performed. The fourth arm is very useful to press the lung parenchyma and innominate vein and to retract the SVC. After all procedures, a utility incision is made to retrieve the tumor specimen. For the retrieval of the tumor, a strong plastic bag is needed. A chest tube is inserted on the R-VATS side.

11.3.2 Posterior Mediastinal Tumor

Neurogenic tumors are the most common posterior mediastinal tumor. Neurogenic tumors located on the mid or lower portion of the thorax are easily excised with VATS or R-VATS. The merit of R-VATS is remarkable during the removal of the neurogenic tumor in the upper portion. Even a posterior tumor in the apex is approachable with a robotic system, saving sympathetic chains. Robotic magnification is likely

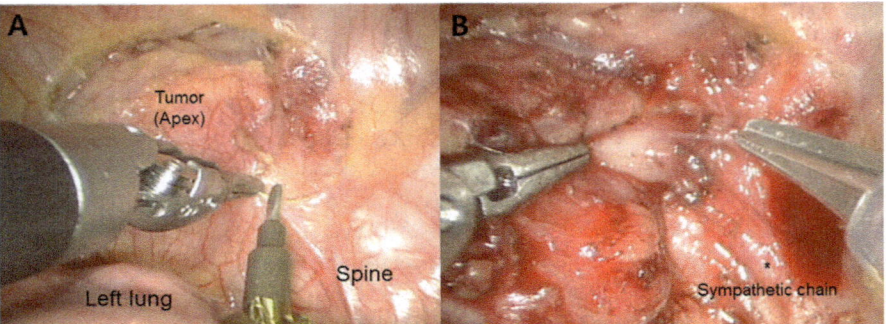

Fig. 11.10 R-VATS excision of a mediastinal tumor in the left apex in a child. In a child, robotic surgery can be performed under bilateral ventilation with intrathoracic CO_2 insufflation

more helpful to prevent Horner's syndrome compared with VATS or an open thoracotomy.

The port placement is the same as that in an R-VATS lobectomy with four arms. R-VATS with three arms can be applied to pediatric cases. R-VATS with three arms with CO_2 insufflation can provide enough space to excise the mediastinal tumor under bilateral lung ventilation with diminished tidal volume (Fig. 11.10).

11.4 Summary

Leonardo da Vinci said, "Simplicity is the ultimate sophistication." During the setup of robotic surgery in the field of thoracic surgery, we have simplified and standardized the port placement and the use of the instruments. Therefore, lung cancer and mediastinal tumors can be managed with the same port placement and instruments. Even for esophageal cancer, a thoracic phase with intrathoracic anastomosis can be performed with the same port placement.

One of the most important aspects of the R-VATS is the depth and accuracy of the hilar and mediastinal nodal dissections. R-VATS provides articulated movement, elimination of physiologic tremor, and a three-dimensional view of the limited space through a small incision. Another strong benefit of robotic surgery is the stable camera platform, which is held by the robotic arm. Because minor movements of the camera can result in image movement, the capacity to provide a steady image is an important benefit of robotic surgery. These merits facilitate LN dissection by enabling more precise instrument movements around the vessels. We found that the dissection of the LNs around major vessels was easier with a magnified three-dimensional view and articulated. These advantages could prevent injury to several nerves, such as the pulmonary and cardiac branches of the vagus nerve. Robotic surgery represents an easy way to expand the indications of MIS towards advanced lung cancer.

From the perspective of the patient, concrete and statistical data are lacking; nevertheless, because the robotic surgeries are performed in a stable setting, postoperative recovery is easier. The magnified operative field and ability to control the surgical view resulted in a low conversion rate related to the experience and dexterity of the surgeon and reduced trauma to the heart and lungs during the robotic surgery, which might be related to the decreased rate of postoperative morbidity.

There is little comparative evidence from randomized controlled trials, and any outcomes from such study designs are affected by variations in surgeon training and experience, which is difficult to assess and adjust for statistically. Consequently, the influence of intra-surgeon technical heterogeneity may outweigh the differences in the surgical approach. However, population-based, observational studies have demonstrated fewer complications for robotic-assisted procedures, such as a pulmonary lobectomy, than those without robotic assistance. The results of this systematic review suggest that R-VATS is feasible and can be performed safely for selected patients in specialized centers [30]. The perioperative outcomes, including postoperative complications, were similar to historical accounts of conventional VATS [14].

In general, robotic surgery has been reported to require more time than thoracoscopic or conventional open surgery. The prolonged operation time is caused by the additional setup time required for the robotic arms. The time spent docking and setting up the robotic arms, which is the main reason for the time delay in other reports, decreases with experience [8, 14, 18]. Robert McKenna suggested that the time limit for the VATS procedure of approximately 3 h in general should be set in advance so that the general anesthesia is not excessive [44]. However, the console time was reduced to less than 3 h after 60 cases based on our series. After achieving the learning curve, the operative times for a robotic lobectomy are comparable with those for a VATS lobectomy.

The lack of tactile feedback could result in excessive pressure and stress on fragile intrathoracic structures. Robotics removes the surgeon from the field and requires a highly trained assistant in the operative theater. These factors necessitate a highly organized and rehearsed approach to the operation, especially in the event of complications such as catastrophic bleeding. In the beginning, we had used three incisions, similar to VATS lobectomy [14]. We used three arms to keep the same number of ports as in VATS lobectomy. However, this approach depends on the experience of the assistant. The use of four arms allows less dependence on the assistant. The role of the assistant is merely to perform the suction, use the endostaplers, and remove the specimen. Four-arm robotic surgery requiring more spatial conception must be performed by a experienced surgeon with the three-arm version of the technique.

Park et al. reported that the cost of open thoracotomy for lung cancer in the USA was high due to the longer hospital stay than that required by VATS or robotic surgery [45]. VATS was the least expensive option. However, this issue depends on each country's insurance system. For example, in Korea, as the reimbursement system is supported by the National Health Insurance system, an open thoracotomy is the least expensive option, despite the extended hospital stay, due to the 95 % reimbursement to cancer patients. The total hospital costs are similar between VATS and robotic surgery, approximately US$11,000. However, there is no reimbursement for the robotic operation from the reimbursement system. Patients who undergo robotic surgery have to pay all costs, which amount to approximately US$10,000. The decision to pursue a particular surgical method is therefore a reflection of socioeconomic status. The excessive costs urge close scrutiny of the benefits of robotic surgery with respect to the patient and the surgeon as well as social and hospital-related considerations.

Robotic surgery is the starting point in the field of thoracic surgery. However, surgeons are enthusiastic about the outstanding merits of the robotic system, which differ from those of VATS. Robot-assisted surgery may provide a good alternative to conventional open or thoracoscopic surgery for lung cancer, provided that the cost-effectiveness and long-term prognosis are confirmed.

Acknowledgments I would like to send a great thanks to my mentor, Dr. Jae Ill Zo for always being in my corner with great support. And, I appreciate all my patients and colleagues for my robotic surgeries.

References

1. Kwoh YS, Hou J, Jonckheere EA, Hayati S (1988) A robot with improved absolute positioning accuracy for CT guided stereotactic brain surgery. IEEE Trans Bio Med Eng 35(2):153–160. doi:10.1109/10.1354
2. Satava RM (2002) Surgical robotics: the early chronicles—a personal historical perspective. Surg Laparosc Endosc Percutan Tech 12(1):6–16
3. Anderson CA, Hellan M, Falebella A, Lau CS, Grannis FW, Kernstine KH (2007) Robotic-assisted lung resection for malignant disease. Innovations 2(5):254–258. doi:10.1097/IMI.0b013e31815e52f1
4. Ashton RC Jr, Connery CP, Swistel DG, DeRose JJ Jr (2003) Robot-assisted lobectomy. J Thorac Cardiovasc Surg 126(1):292–293
5. Augustin F, Bodner J, Wykypiel H, Schwinghammer C, Schmid T (2011) Initial experience with robotic lung lobectomy: report of two different approaches. Surg Endosc 25(1):108–113. doi:10.1007/s00464-010-1138-3
6. Bodner J, Wykypiel H, Wetscher G, Schmid T (2004) First experiences with the *da Vinci*™ operating robot in thoracic surgery. Eur J Cardiothorac Surg 25(5):844–851. doi:10.1016/j.ejcts.2004.02.001
7. Braumann C, Jacobi CA, Menenakos C, Ismail M, Rueckert JC, Mueller JM (2008) Robotic-assisted laparoscopic and thoracoscopic surgery with the *da Vinci* system: a 4-year experience in a single institution. Surg Laparosc Endosc Percutan Tech 18(3):260–266. doi:10.1097/SLE.0b013e31816f85e5
8. Cerfolio RJ, Bryant AS, Skylizard L, Minnich DJ (2011) Initial consecutive experience of completely portal robotic pulmonary resection with 4 arms. J Thorac Cardiovasc Surg 142(4):740–746. doi:10.1016/j.jtcvs.2011.07.022
9. Dylewski MR, Ohaeto AC, Pereira JF (2011) Pulmonary resection using a total endoscopic robotic video-assisted approach. Semin Thorac Cardiovasc Surg 23(1):36–42. doi:10.1053/j.semtcvs.2011.01.005

10. Gharagozloo F, Margolis M, Tempesta B (2008) Robot-assisted thoracoscopic lobectomy for early-stage lung cancer. Ann Thorac Surg 85(6):1880–1885. doi:10.1016/j.athoracsur.2008.02.085, Discussion 1885-1886
11. Gharagozloo F, Margolis M, Tempesta B, Strother E, Najam F (2009) Robot-assisted lobectomy for early-stage lung cancer: report of 100 consecutive cases. Ann Thorac Surg 88(2):380–384. doi:10.1016/j.athoracsur.2009.04.039
12. Giulianotti PC, Buchs NC, Caravaglios G, Bianco FM (2010) Robot-assisted lung resection: outcomes and technical details. Interact Cardiovasc Thorac Surg 11(4):388–392. doi:10.1510/icvts.2010.239541
13. Giulianotti PC, Coratti A, Angelini M, Sbrana F, Cecconi S, Balestracci T, Caravaglios G (2003) Robotics in general surgery: personal experience in a large community hospital. Arch Surg 138(7):777–784. doi:10.1001/archsurg.138.7.777
14. Jang HJ, Lee HS, Park SY, Zo JI (2011) Comparison of the early robot-assisted lobectomy experience to video-assisted thoracic surgery lobectomy for lung cancer: a single-institution case series matching study. Innovations 6(5):305–310. doi:10.1097/IMI.0b013e3182378b4c
15. Kernstine KH, Anderson CA, Falabella A (2008) Robotic lobectomy. Oper Tech Thorac Cardiovasc Surg 13(3):204.e1–204.e23
16. Melfi FM, Menconi GF, Mariani AM, Angeletti CA (2002) Early experience with robotic technology for thoracoscopic surgery. Eur J Cardiothorac Surg 21(5):864–868
17. Park BJ, Flores RM, Rusch VW (2006) Robotic assistance for video-assisted thoracic surgical lobectomy: technique and initial results. J Thorac Cardiovasc Surg 131(1):54–59. doi:10.1016/j.jtcvs.2005.07.031
18. Veronesi G, Galetta D, Maisonneuve P, Melfi F, Schmid RA, Borri A, Vannucci F, Spaggiari L (2010) Four-arm robotic lobectomy for the treatment of early-stage lung cancer. J Thorac Cardiovasc Surg 140(1):19–25. doi:10.1016/j.jtcvs.2009.10.025
19. Mohr FW (2011) Pioneer in cardiac surgery. Circulation 123:f74
20. Ginsberg RJ, Rubinstein LV (1995) Randomized trial of lobectomy versus limited resection for T1 N0 non-small cell lung cancer. Lung cancer study group. Ann Thorac Surg 60(3):615–622, Discussion 622–613
21. Swanson SJ, Herndon JE II, D'Amico TA, Demmy TL, McKenna RJ Jr, Green MR, Sugarbaker DJ (2007) Video-assisted thoracic surgery lobectomy: report of CALGB 39802—a prospective, multi-institution feasibility study. J Clin Oncol 25(31):4993–4997
22. Rueth NM, Andrade RS (2010) Is VATS lobectomy better: perioperatively, biologically and oncologically? Ann Thorac Surg 89:S2107–2111. doi:10.1016/j.athoracsur.2010.03.020
23. Farjah F, Wood DE, Mulligan MS, Krishnadasan B, Heagerty PJ, Symons RG, Flum DR (2009) Safety and efficacy of video-assisted versus conventional lung resection for lung cancer. J Thorac Cardiovasc Surg 137(6):1415–1421. doi:10.1016/j.jtcvs.2008.11 035
24. Flores RM, Alam N (2008) Video-assisted thoracic surgery lobectomy (VATS), open thoracotomy, and the robot for lung cancer. Ann Thorac Surg 85(2):S710–715. doi:10.1016/j.athoracsur.2007.09.055
25. Grogan EL, Jones DR (2008) VATS lobectomy is better than open thoracotomy: what is the evidence for short-term outcomes? Thorac Surg Clin 18(3):249–258. doi:10.1016/j.thorsurg.2008.04.007
26. Petersen RP, Pham D, Burfeind WR, Hanish SI, Toloza EM, Harpole DH Jr, D'Amico TA (2007) Thoracoscopic lobectomy facilitates the delivery of chemotherapy after resection for lung cancer. Ann Thorac Surg 83(4):1245–1249. doi:10.1016/j.athoracsur.2006.12.029, Discussion 1250
27. Whitson BA, D'Cunha J, Andrade RS, Kelly RF, Groth SS, Wu B, Miller JS, Kratzke RA, Maddaus MA (2008) Thoracoscopic versus thoracotomy approaches to lobectomy: differential impairment of cellular immunity. Ann Thorac Surg 86(6):1735–1744. doi:10.1016/j.athoracsur.2008.07.001
28. Yan TD, Black D, Bannon PG, McCaughan BC (2009) Systematic review and meta-analysis of randomized and nonrandomized trials on safety and efficacy of video-assisted thoracic surgery

lobectomy for early-stage non-small-cell lung cancer. J Clin Oncol 27(15):2553–2562. doi:10.1200/JCO.2008.18.2733
29. Boffa DJ, Allen MS, Grab JD, Gaissert HA, Harpole DH, Wright CD (2008) Data from the society of thoracic surgeons general thoracic surgery database: the surgical management of primary lung tumors. J Thorac Cardiovasc Surg 135(2):247–254. doi:10.1016/j.jtcvs.2007.07.060
30. Cao C, Manganas C, Ang SC, Yan TD (2012) A systematic review and meta-analysis on pulmonary resections by robotic video-assisted thoracic surgery. Ann Cardiothorac Surg 1(1):3–10. doi:10.3978/j.issn.2225-319X.2012.04.03
31. Lee HS, Jang HJ (2012) Thoracoscopic mediastinal lymph node dissection for lung cancer. Semin Thorac Cardiovasc Surg 24(2):131–141. doi:10.1053/j.semtcvs.2012.02.004
32. Darling GE, Allen MS, Decker PA, Ballman K, Malthaner RA, Inculet RI, Jones DR, McKenna RJ, Landreneau RJ, Rusch VW (2011) Randomized trial of mediastinal lymph node sampling versus complete lymphadenectomy during pulmonary resection in the patient with N0 or N1 (less than hilar) non-small cell carcinoma: results of the American college of surgery oncology group Z0030 trial. J Thorac Cardiovasc Surg 141(3):662–670. doi:10.1016/j.jtcvs.2010.11.008
33. Izbicki J, Thetter O, Habekost M, Karg O, Passlick B, Kubuschok B, Busch C, Haeussinger K, Knoefel W, Pantel K (2005) Radical systematic mediastinal lymphadenectomy in non-small cell lung cancer: a randomized controlled trial. Br J Surg 81(2):229–235
34. Keller SM, Adak S, Wagner H, Johnson DH (2000) Mediastinal lymph node dissection improves survival in patients with stages II and IIIa non-small cell lung cancer. Eastern cooperative oncology group. Ann Thorac Surg 70(2):358–365, Discussion 365–356
35. Park JS, Kim K, Choi MS, Chang SW, Han WS (2011) Video-assisted thoracic surgery (VATS) lobectomy for pathologic stage I non-small cell lung cancer: a comparative study with thoracotomy lobectomy. Korean J Thorac Cardiovasc Surg 44(1):32–38. doi:10.5090/kjtcs.2011.44.1.32
36. Sagawa M, Sato M, Sakurada A, Matsumura Y, Endo C, Handa M, Kondo T (2002) A prospective trial of systematic nodal dissection for lung cancer by video-assisted thoracic surgery: can it be perfect? Ann Thorac Surg 73(3):900–904
37. Watanabe A, Koyanagi T, Ohsawa H, Mawatari T, Nakashima S, Takahashi N, Sato H, Abe T (2005) Systematic node dissection by VATS is not inferior to that through an open thoracotomy: a comparative clinicopathologic retrospective study. Surgery 138(3):510–517
38. Park BJ, Melfi F, Mussi A, Maisonneuve P, Spaggiari L, Da Silva RK, Veronesi G (2012) Robotic lobectomy for non-small cell lung cancer (NSCLC): long-term oncologic results. J Thorac Cardiovasc Surg 143(2):383–389. doi:10.1016/j.jtcvs.2011.10.055
39. Park BJ (2012) Robotic lobectomy for non-small cell lung cancer (NSCLC): multi-center registry study of long-term oncologic results. Ann Cardiothorac Surg 1(1):24–26. doi:10.3978/j.issn2225-319X.2012.04
40. Goldstraw P, Crowley J, Chansky K, Giroux DJ, Groome PA, Rami-Porta R, Postmus PE, Rusch V, Sobin L, International Association for the Study of Lung Cancer International Staging C, Participating I (2007) The IASLC lung cancer staging project: proposals for the revision of the TNM stage groupings in the forthcoming (seventh) edition of the TNM Classification of malignant tumours. J Thorac Oncol: Official Publication of the International Association for the Study of Lung Cancer 2(8):706–714. doi:10.1097/JTO.0b013e31812f3c1a
41. Toker A, Sonett J, Zielinski M, Rea F, Tomulescu V, Detterbeck FC (2011) Standard terms, definitions, and policies for minimally invasive resection of thymoma. J Thorac Oncol 6(7 Suppl 3):S1739–1742. doi:10.1097/JTO.0b013e31821ea553
42. Marulli G, Rea F, Melfi F, Schmid TA, Ismail M, Fanucchi O, Augustin F, Swierzy M, Di Chiara F, Mussi A, Rueckert JC (2012) Robot-aided thoracoscopic thymectomy for early-stage thymoma: a multicenter European study. J Thorac Cardiovasc Surg 144(5):1125–1130. doi:10.1016/j.jtcvs.2012.07.082

43. Toker A, Erus S, Ozkan B, Ziyade S, Tanju S (2011) Does a relationship exist between the number of thoracoscopic thymectomies performed and the learning curve for thoracoscopic resection of thymoma in patients with myasthenia gravis? Interact Cardiovasc Thorac Surg 12 (2):152–155. doi:10.1510/icvts.2010.254599, Epub 2010 Nov 9
44. McKenna RJ Jr (2008) Complications and learning curves for video-assisted thoracic surgery lobectomy. Thorac Surg Clin 18(3):275–280. doi:10.1016/j.thorsurg.2008.04.004
45. Park BJ, Flores RM (2008) Cost comparison of robotic, video-assisted thoracic surgery and thoracotomy approaches to pulmonary lobectomy. Thorac Surg Clin 18(3):297–300. doi:10.1016/j.thorsurg.2008.05.003, vii

Robot-Assisted Thyroidectomy

12

Norihiko Ishikawa

12.1 History of Thyroidectomy

Thyroidectomy is the goal of the initial therapy of thyroid cancer, and it is performed to remove the primary tumor that has extended beyond the thyroid capsule and the involved cervical lymph nodes. Surgery is the most important treatment to affect the prognosis while radioactive iodine treatment, thyroid-stimulating hormone suppression, and external beam irradiation each play adjunctive roles in many patients. Most departments of surgery follow the standard technique. The principles of safe and efficient thyroid surgery have been established since the early nineteenth century and the "10 commandments" of thyroid surgery are universally accepted as the standard for traditional open thyroidectomy [3]. A 5- to 6-cm-long Kocher incision is made in the neck, flaps are raised, and the strap muscles are divided transversely.

In 1997, two brief reports of endoscopic thyroid surgery procedures were published, and Gagner made the first report of endoscopic parathyroid surgery in 1996 [4]. With the tendency to develop shorter incisions, an endoscopic approach has been applied to surgery of both the thyroid and parathyroid glands. These endoscopic techniques attempt to minimize the extent of dissection, improving cosmesis, reducing postoperative pain, shortening hospital stay, and enhancing postoperative recovery. The most common minimally invasive technique is minimally invasive video-assisted thyroidectomy (MIVAT) [5]. On the other hand, the extracervical approach is considered endoscopic instead of MIVAT because incisions are made distant from the neck, so that the procedure requires more extensive tissue dissections [6]. These approaches have been adopted more often

N. Ishikawa (✉)
Department of General and Cardiothoracic Surgery, Kanazawa University,
13-1 Takaramachi, Kanazawa, Ishikawa 920-8641, Japan
e-mail: iskwnrhk@gmail.com

in Asian countries, and an increasing number of different endoscopic techniques has been described [7, 8]. Robotic thyroidectomy is a new approach that offers many benefits, mostly overcoming the limitations of standard endoscopic surgery [9].

12.2 Minimally Invasive Video-Assisted Thyroidectomy (MIVAT)

The endoscopic lateral cervical approach and MIVAT were developed in the late 1990s, and these minimally invasive techniques have been thoroughly researched since the first description of the technique by Ganger et al. [4]. MIVAT for thyroid tumor was described for the first time by Miccoli [5, 8, 10–15]. These procedures are categorized as cervical approaches.

Two 2.5-mm and one 10-mm trocars are inserted along the anterior border of the sternocleidomastoid muscle on the side of resection. Excellent visualization of the recurrent laryngeal nerve (RLN) and parathyroid glands is possible with magnification by the endoscope. However, this technique is limited to unilateral thyroid resection, and its application in thyroid cancer surgery is restricted to small papillary thyroid carcinoma. The procedure is performed under endoscopic view with the operating space maintained by external retraction (Fig. 12.1a). The MIVAT technique follows the same principles as standard thyroidectomy [10]; the main difference is that the incision is much shorter (1.5–2 cm). With improvements in techniques, MIVAT has become increasingly adopted for low-to-intermediate risk differentiated thyroid cancer [16]. In addition, it has been shown that a concomitant central neck dissection is technically feasible in MIVAT during initial total thyroidectomy [17]. However, MIVAT for thyroid cancers warrants a more strict set of indications.

12.3 Endoscopic Thyroidectomy

Compared with conventional open surgery, endoscopic surgery can greatly reduce operation wounds, lessen postoperative pain, shorten hospital stays, and improve cosmetic outcomes. Endoscopic technique has been used in all surgical fields for more than 20 years.

After Gagner's report, the use of an endoscopic parathyroidectomy procedure with CO_2 insufflation has become widespread [4, 18–20]. Currently, depending on the institute where the surgery is performed, various incision sites are used, including the neck [21–23], chest wall [24–26], axilla [27], breast [28], and submandibular [29] area. In creating the working space, both CO_2 insufflation and gasless lifting methods have been applied.

The efficacy and safety of endoscopic thyroidectomy have been verified in quite large multi-institutional series [30], and it has been demonstrated that VAT has some advantages over traditional thyroidectomy in terms of cosmetic results and postoperative pain [31]. Lombardi et al. also proved the safety of endoscopic

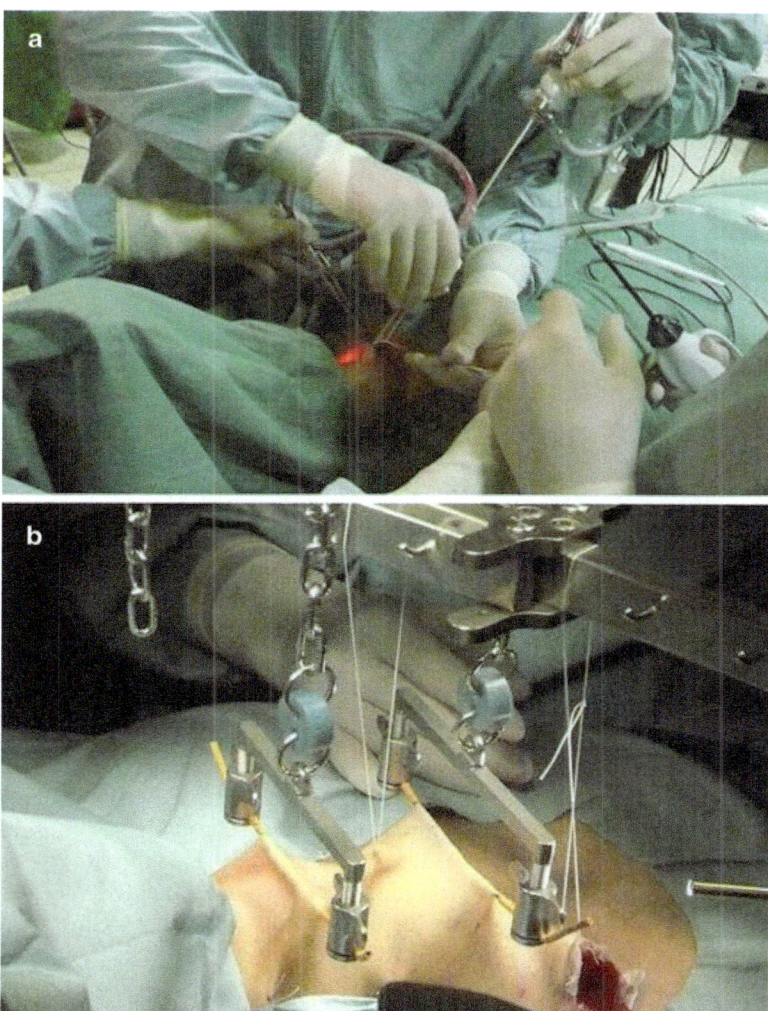

Fig. 12.1 (a) Intraoperative view of the minimally invasive video-assisted thyroidectomy. (b) Picture of an anterior neck-lift method in endoscopic thyroidectomy

thyroidectomy versus the traditional procedure [14]. Significant advantages of endoscopic thyroidectomy over open thyroidectomy in terms of less painful postoperative course and better cosmetic result have also been confirmed [5–7, 10–15, 31]. A randomized, controlled trial was conducted by Jiang et al. [32] to evaluate the technical feasibility of endoscopic thyroidectomy, and the trial found it to be as safe as open surgery with the same complication rates. The advantage of BAET was patient satisfaction with the cosmetic results. Disadvantages included longer operation time and higher cost. The accepted indications for endoscopic thyroidectomy are unilateral or bilateral benign lesions. However, for experienced surgeons, the inclusion criteria for thyroid carcinoma should be papillary microcarcinoma (<1 cm) without signs of capsule invasion and involvement of the central or lateral compartment lymph nodes.

12.3.1 Breast Approach

The first cases of this procedure were reported in 1998 by Ishii et al. [33]. The aim of this technique was to avoid the presence of any scars in the neck. The two working ports are inserted through circumareolar incisions on both breasts. The camera port (1.5–2.0 cm) is placed over the right parasternal region. A subcutaneous tunnel is created using blunt dissection, and a subplatysmal space is created. Insufflation with CO_2 is started to ready the subplatysmal working space. Working instruments are introduced until the thyroid bed is reached under endoscopic vision. From that point, the steps of the procedure are the same as the standard classical technique, but all are performed endoscopically by first working in one pole and then the other.

12.3.2 Anterior Chest Approach

Shimizu developed a totally gasless endoscopic surgical technique using an anterior neck skin-lifting method for thyroid and parathyroid diseases in March 1998 [23] and performed more than 200 minimally invasive endoscopic thyroid operations [26]. This technique involves an approximately 4-cm oblique incision on the tumor side of the chest wall, 3 cm below the clavicle for insertion of an ultrasonically activated scalpel and a grasper. Then, a 2-cm incision is made in the lateral neck on the tumor side. To create a working space, two pieces of 1.2-mm-diameter Kirschner wire are horizontally inserted through the subcutaneous layer of developed flap of the anterior neck skin (Fig. 12.1b).

12.3.3 Transaxillary Approach

Ikeda et al. first described these approaches by placing three ports in the axilla with low-pressure CO_2 insufflation to maintain the surgical field. Although the cosmetic results were excellent, the procedure was technically demanding and time consuming because of unintentional easy gas leakage and frequent interference of the surgical instruments in the small available space [34]. Kang et al. modified this technique by making this approach gasless with the space maintained by a specially designed skin-lifting external retractor [35]. In this approach, a subcutaneous space was created from the 4- to 5-cm incision in the axilla to the thyroid gland. To avoid the problem of interference of instruments, an additional 5-mm port was made in the chest area for medial retraction of the thyroid gland. To further increase the degree of angulations and freedom of interference among instruments, a combined axillo-breast approach was developed using two circumareolar trocars in the breast and a single trocar in the ipsilateral axilla. This approach was later modified using bilateral axillary ports to allow better exposure to both sides of the thyroid compartment. This approach is now known as the bilateral axillo-breast approach (BABA). Despite the extensive tissue dissection, when compared with the conventional open approach, BABA has been shown to have similar results in terms of transient hypocalcemia, bleeding, permanent RLN paralysis, and length of hospital stay [36]. These gasless transaxillary approaches and BABA will be major basic procedures for robot-assisted thyroidectomy.

12.4 Robotic Thyroidectomy

The learning curve of endoscopic surgery is especially long, and robotic surgery is being increasingly accepted to make difficult conventional endoscopic procedures easier and to improve surgical efficiency and efficacy. In the field of thyroid surgery, the initial application of robotic surgery was simple lobectomy for goiter in 2005, and it has been successfully extended to total thyroidectomy combined with cervical lymph node dissection for thyroid cancer [37–40]. All-robotic thyroidectomy has been reported in the use of the da Vinci surgical system (Intuitive Surgical Inc., Sunnyvale, CA, USA). Not only partial thyroidectomy but also cervical lymph node dissection for thyroid cancer can be performed with conventional endoscopic surgery [37]. However, there is no natural space, and the artificial operation space is relatively narrow in endoscopic neck surgery. The conventional endoscopic thyroid surgery is still not widely accepted for several reasons: two-dimensional images, inflexible instruments, prolonged learning curve, and difficult manipulation of the RLN and parathyroid gland. In the robotic surgical view, the important structures such as the RLN and parathyroid gland can be simply identified and manipulated under the 3-D magnified view [38–44], and cervical lymph node dissection of the suprasternal fossa, which is difficult to reach for the conventional endoscopic surgery, can be performed easily using the flexible robotic instruments. Many studies have suggested that robot-assisted endoscopic thyroid surgery is safe and feasible for most patients with thyroid carcinoma, since precise lymph node dissection and satisfactory cosmetic results can be achieved with robotic technology.

12.5 Transaxillary Approach

Chung et al. at Yonsei University College of Medicine (Seoul) reported gasless transaxillary thyroidectomy using the da Vinci since late 2007 [45–47].

Surgical procedure: With the patient placed supine under general anesthesia, the neck is slightly extended, and the lesion-side arm is raised and fixed. A 5- to 6-cm-long vertical skin incision is then made in the axilla, and a subcutaneous

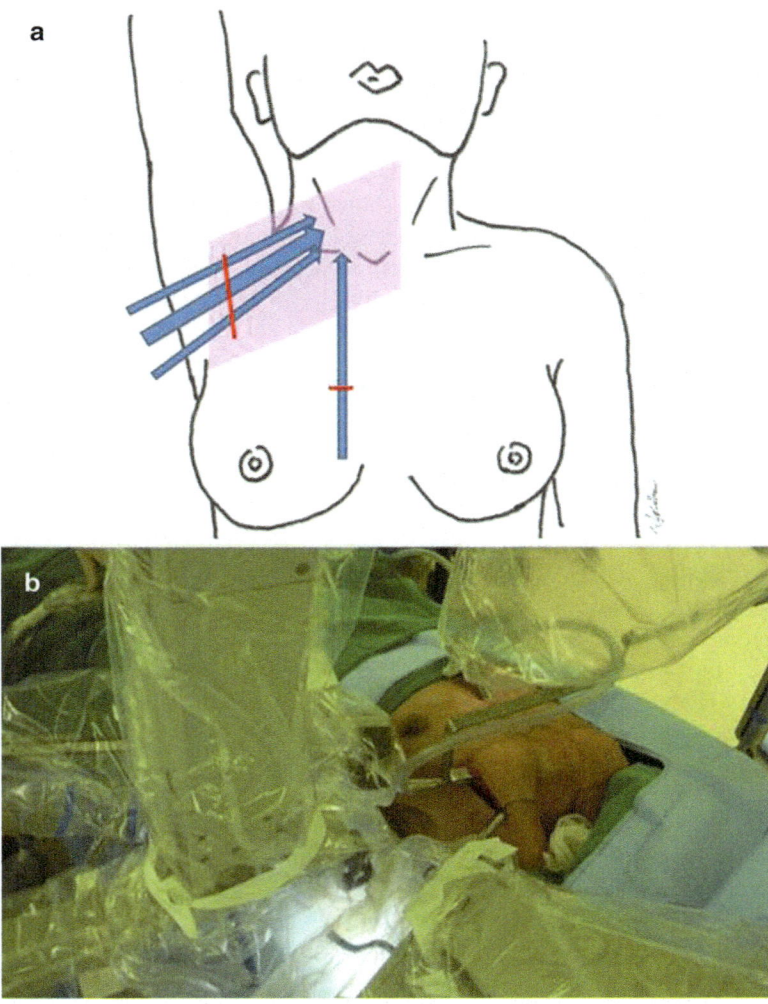

Fig. 12.2 Robot-assisted thyroidectomy using transaxillary approach. (**a**) Proposal plans of dissection. The *pink zone* represents the area of frap dissection. (**b**) Operative view

skin flap is dissected over the anterior surface of the pectoralis major muscle and clavicle under direct vision (Fig. 12.2a). After exposing the medial border of the sternocleidomastoid muscle, the dissection is approached through the avascular space of the sternocleidomastoid muscle branches (between the sternal and clavicular heads) and beneath the strap muscle until the contralateral lobe of the thyroid is exposed. To maintain the working space, an external retractor is then inserted through the skin incision in the axilla and raised using a lifting device (Fig. 12.3a). A second skin incision (0.8-cm long) is made on the medial side of the anterior chest wall to insert the fourth robot arm, 2 cm superiorly and 6–8 cm medially from

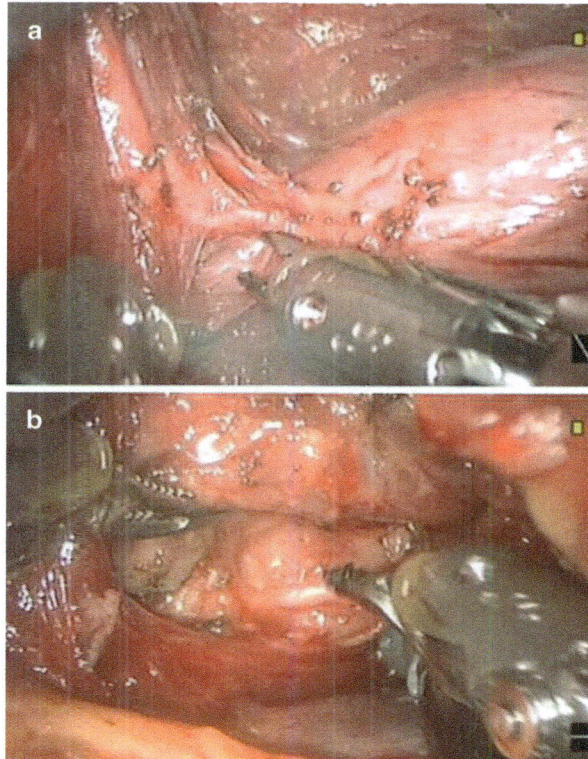

Fig. 12.3 Surgical procedure for the transaxillary approach. (**a**) Ligation of the superior laryngeal artery. (**b**) Identification of the recurrent laryngeal nerve

the nipple. The other three arms are inserted through the axillary incision (Fig. 12.2b). The operation proceeds in the same manner as conventional open thyroidectomy. Under endoscopic guidance, the upper pole of the thyroid is drawn downward and medially, and the superior thyroid vessels are identified and individually divided close to the thyroid gland to avoid injuring the external branch of the superior laryngeal nerve (Fig. 12.3). The thyroid gland is then pulled in a superior and medial direction, and the central compartment node dissection is started from the common carotid artery to the inferior thyroid artery superiorly and to the substernal notch inferiorly. After exposing the common carotid artery and inferior thyroid artery, soft tissues and lymph nodes in the pretracheal area are detached from cervical thymic tissues and dissected to the substernal notch. Careful dissection is performed to identify the inferior thyroid artery and the RLN. During this procedure, the paraesophageal lymph nodes are detached from the tracheoesophageal groove. The inferior thyroid artery is then divided close to the thyroid gland, and the whole cervical course of the RLN is traced. The superior parathyroid gland is identified and left intact. The thyroid gland is dissected from the trachea and the prelaryngeal lymph nodes with the pyramidal lobe are also detached from the thyroid cartilage. Contralateral thyroidectomy is performed using the same

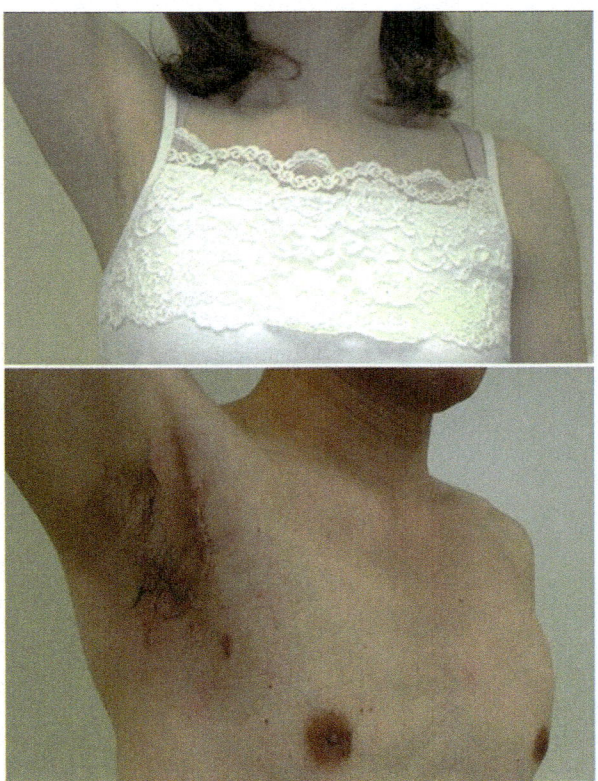

Fig. 12.4 Postoperative picture

method with medial traction of the thyroid. A closed-suction drain is inserted through a separate skin incision under the axillary skin incision. The wound is closed cosmetically.

This procedure has several advantages for thyroidectomy. First, the upper and lower poles of the thyroid and neck lymph nodes can be easily revealed and manipulated. Second, the parathyroid glands and RLN can be directly exposed in the lateral view; thus, ipsilateral neck lymph node dissection can be safely performed without injuries to important tissues and organs. Third, a stable and plain working space established with the gasless method can be maintained by continuous negative pressure suction of the air and blood. Also, postoperative hypoesthesia and fibrotic contracture in the anterior neck area can be effectively avoided because no anterior neck flap dissection is required (Fig. 12.4). The limitation of this approach is the difficulty of exposing and resecting the contralateral thyroid lobe through a unilateral axillary approach.

The indications for this procedure are minimally invasive follicular thyroid carcinoma 4 cm or less in diameter or papillary thyroid carcinoma 2 cm or less in diameter [45–47], but in the future, the application of robotic technology in endoscopic thyroid surgeries could overcome the limitations of conventional endoscopic surgeries in the surgical management of selected patients with thyroid cancer. Contraindications to robotic thyroidectomy include previous neck operations; prior vocal fold paralysis or a history of voice or laryngeal disease requiring therapy; malignancy with extrathyroid invasion; multiple neck node metastases; perinodal infiltration at a metastatic lymph node; distant metastasis; and a lesion located in the thyroid dorsal area that can lead to a possible injury of the trachea, esophagus, or RLN during the procedure. Previous studies compiled the indications and limitations of the technique and showed that robot-assisted thyroidectomy is as effective and safe as traditional thyroidectomy. Robotic thyroidectomy using a transaxillary approach leaves the patient with an incision scar in the axilla that is completely covered by the patient's arm when in a natural position, which makes the small central incision almost invisible. Previous studies have reported that patients who underwent thyroidectomy by the transaxillary approach reported mild pain or discomfort in the neck and the anterior chest wall [34, 48, 49]. This may be caused by the extended dissection from the axilla to the neck.

A prospective study of this procedure using the da Vinci surgical system for 338 patients with thyroid tumor was performed by the Yonsei group. In this study, thyroidectomy and central neck lymph node dissection were successfully completed using a gasless, transaxillary approach. For radical neck lymph node dissection, conventional endoscopic surgery has usually been performed as in thyroidectomy for low-risk thyroid cancer patients without detectable nodal disease. However, with the aid of robotic surgical systems, the indications for endoscopic thyroid surgery have been extended, and the same operative outcomes as with open surgery can be achieved when dissecting the lateral neck lymph nodes. Furthermore, Kang et al. reported robotic modified radical thyroidectomy, including total thyroidectomy and central and lateral neck lymph node dissection, in 33 patients with thyroid carcinoma and lymph node metastases, and there were no serious postoperative complications such as RLN injury or hypoparathyroidism [50]. The da Vinci surgical system can access the lateral neck area, such as the internal jugular vein joining the subclavian vein or the uppermost region of level II, regions inaccessible to the conventional endoscopic instruments. Based on their experience, robot-assisted modified radical neck dissection should be viewed as an acceptable alternative method in patients with low-risk, well-differentiated thyroid cancer with lateral neck node metastasis.

12.6 Bilateral Axillo-Breast Approach (BABA)

Surgical procedure: Under general anesthesia, the patient is placed in the supine position with the arms tucked close to the side. Epinephrine solution is injected into the subcutaneous space of both breasts and the subplatysmal space in the neck to help dissection and reduce bleeding. Two 5-mm circumareolar incisions, a 12-mm axillary incision at the lesion side, and a 5-mm axillary incision at the opposite side are made (Fig. 12.5). The flaps are bluntly dissected with a vascular tunneler. After blunt dissection, ports are inserted through each incision, and the flaps are

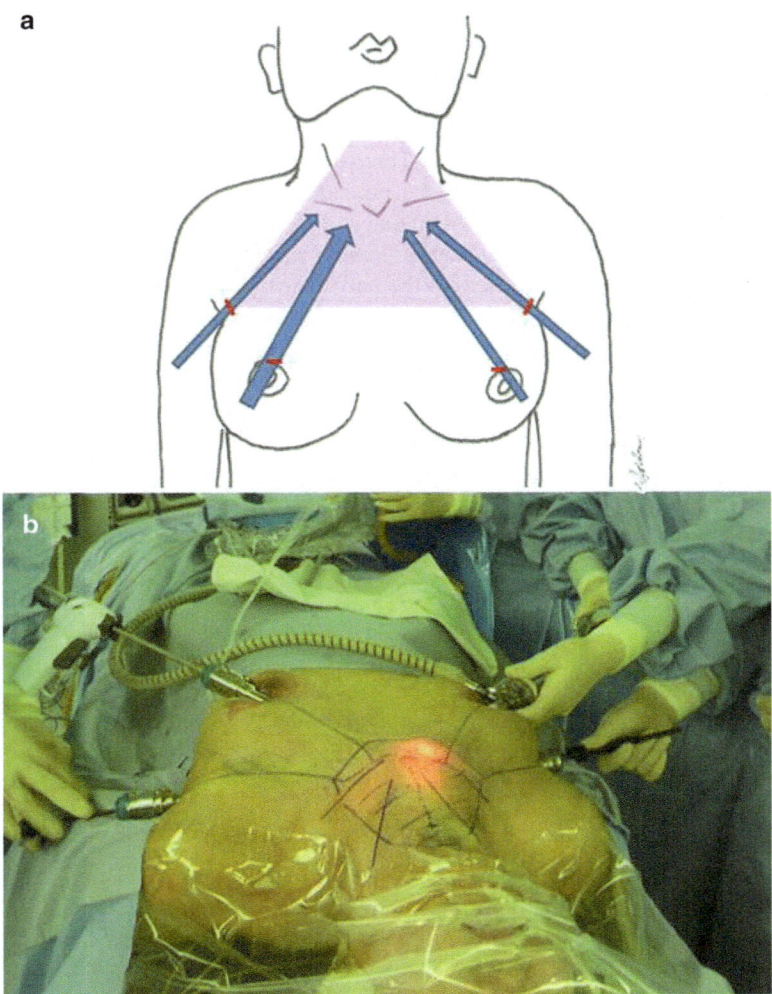

Fig. 12.5 Robot-assisted thyroidectomy using bilateral axillo-breast approach. (**a**) Proposal plans of dissection. The *pink zone* represents the area of frap dissection. (**b**) Operative view

insufflated with CO_2 at 5–6-mmHg pressure with a flow rate of 2 L/min (20–30 mL/kg/min). The flaps are extended with ultrasonic shears from the level of the thyroid cartilage to the sternal notch and laterally to the medial border of each sternocleidomastoid muscle. A midline division of the strap muscles is made from the level of the thyroid cartilage to the sternal notch, and the isthmus of the thyroid gland is divided using ultrasonic shears. A snake-shaped retractor is used to retract the strap muscles laterally. The inferolateral side of the thyroid gland is carefully dissected to find the RLN and the inferior parathyroid gland. After identification of the RLN, the plane just superficial to the nerve is delineated with an endo-dissector, and Berry's ligament is divided using ultrasonic shears. The thyroid specimen is pulled out through the 12-mm axillary incision using an endoplastic bag. In cases of selective lateral neck dissection, the sternocleidomastoid muscle is retracted laterally with the snake-shaped retractor, and the lateral compartment is dissected with ultrasonic shears or by electrocautery. Meticulous hemostasis is performed, and the strap muscles are re-approximated with absorbable sutures. One or two closed-suction drains are inserted into the operative bed through each axillary incision. Surgical brassieres are applied to provide compression of the flaps.

Robot-assisted BABA allows an open vision of important anatomical landmarks such as the trachea, RLN, and parathyroid glands, enabling the surgeons to perform a bilateral total thyroidectomy conveniently and effectively avoid serious operative complications. Lee et al. performed robotic total thyroidectomy and central neck lymph node dissection in a gas-filled working space for 109 patients with differentiated thyroid cancer through BABA, and they reported that the gas-filled, robot-assisted BABA surgery yielded excellent cosmetic outcomes, suggesting that this technique could also be a suitable operative alternative for low-risk patients with thyroid carcinoma [51].

Recently, Singer et al. explored robotic thyroidectomy via a facelift incision in 11 fresh human cadavers and refined a reproducible surgical protocol. In summary, among the various endoscopic approaches, the transaxillary approach is superior in operation time and range of lymph node dissection, while the BABA approach is superior in the thoroughness of thyroidectomy [52]. These differences may be due to the surgeons' proficiency in surgical technique as well as the limitations of the specific operative approach.

Robotic thyroidectomy was developed at Yonsei University, Korea, and several robotic procedures were developed in the Korean institute. Korea is today the country where robotic thyroidectomy is seeing the most use. The Korean group reported a multi-institutional analysis of robotic thyroidectomy compared with endoscopic thyroidectomy [53]. These studies suggest that robotic thyroidectomy has overcome some of the technical limitations associated with conventional endoscopic procedures, with reduced operation times and increased lymph node retrieval. Moreover, we found that the learning curve for robotic thyroidectomy was shorter than that for endoscopic thyroidectomy. Lee also reported that robotic thyroidectomy is superior to endoscopic thyroidectomy in terms of operation time, lymph node retrieval, and the learning curve [54].

However, Yoo reported that robotic thyroidectomy had disadvantages over endoscopic thyroidectomy due to lengthier duration, higher cost, longer drainage, and no improvements in oncologic outcomes and complication rates.

Compared with open surgery, Yi reported the technical and oncologic safety of robotic thyroidectomy [55]. Lee recommended robotic thyroidectomy for several distinct advantages, including its very good to excellent cosmetic result, reduced postoperative neck discomfort, and fewer swallowing symptoms [56]. On the other hand, Perrier's opinion of robot-assisted thyroidectomy is negative for several reasons [57]. Ideal candidates for robot-assisted thyroidectomy were those with a small body habitus like Asian patients but not North American patients, and it was not suitable for patients with known thyroiditis, large nodules, goiter, hyperthyroidism, Graves' disease, or cancer. Furthermore, Perrier mentioned that an additional incision for larger patients in the breast or parasternal region would obscure tissue in future mammograms and could cause additional disruption in breast sensation.

12.7 Conclusion

Robotic technologies have undoubtedly had a positive impact on the surgical management of thyroid cancer. The application of endoscopic visualization of the thyroid gland has allowed surgeons to perform safe surgery from extracervical skin incisions. Although short-term outcome studies in several robotic procedures demonstrated technical and oncologic safety and excellent cosmetic results for differentiated thyroid cancer, no prospective trials comparing the clinical results of robotic, conventional endoscopic, and open thyroidectomy have been described. If further prospective randomized trials confirm the advantages of robotic thyroidectomy compared with conventional endoscopic and open surgery, this technique may become the preferred option for most patients undergoing surgery for thyroid cancer.

References

1. Hegedus L (2004) Clinical practice. The thyroid nodule. N Engl J Med 351:1764–1771
2. Hay ID, Bergstralh EJ, Goellner JR, Ebersold JR, Grant CS (1993) Predicting outcome in papillary thyroid carcinoma: development of a reliable prognostic scoring system in a cohort of 1779 patients surgically treated at one institution during 1940 through 1989. Surgery 114:1050–1057
3. Hobbs CGL, Watkinson JC (2007) Thyroidectomy. Surgery 25:474–478
4. Gagner M (1996) Endoscopic subtotal parathyroidectomy in patients with primary hyperparathyroidism. Br J Surg 83:875
5. Miccoli P, Berti P, Conte M, Bendinelli C, Marcocci C (1999) Minimally invasive surgery for thyroid small nodules: preliminary report. J Endocrinol Invest 22:849–851
6. Henry JF (2008) Minimally invasive thyroid and parathyroid surgery is not a question of length of the incision. Langenbecks Arch Surg 393:621–626
7. Slotema ET, Sebag F, Henry JF (2008) What is the evidence for endoscopic thyroidectomy in the management of benign thyroid disease? World J Surg 32:1325–1332
8. Miccoli P, Minuto MN, Berti P, Materazzi G (2009) Update on the diagnosis and treatment of differentiated thyroid cancer. Q J Nucl Med Mol Imaging 53:465–472
9. Perrier ND, Randolph GW, Inabnet WB, Marple BF, VanHeerden J, Kuppersmith RB (2010) Robotic thyroidectomy: a framework for new technology assessment and safe implementation. Thyroid 20:1327–1332
10. Timon C, Rafferty M (2008) Minimally invasive video-assisted thyroidectomy (MIVAT): technique, advantages, and disadvantages. Oper Tech Otolaryngol Head Neck Surg 19:8–14
11. Ruggieri M, Straniero A, Maiuolo A, Pacini FM, Chatelou E, Batori M, D'Armiento M, Fumarola A, Gargiulo P, Genderini M (2007) The minimally invasive surgical approach in thyroid diseases. Minerva Chir 62:309–314

12. Miccoli P, Materazzi G, Berti P (2010) Minimally invasive thyroidectomy in the treatment of well differentiated thyroid cancers: indications and limits. Curr Opin Otolaryngol Head Neck Surg 18:114–118
13. El-Labban GM (2009) Minimally invasive video-assisted thyroidectomy versus conventional thyroidectomy: a single-blinded, randomized controlled clinical trial. J Minim Access Surg 5:97–102
14. Ombardi CP, Raffaelli M, Princi P, Lulli P, Rossi ED, Fadda G, Bellantone R (2005) Safety of video-assisted thyroidectomy versus conventional surgery. Head Neck 27:58–64
15. Mamais C, Charaklias N, Pothula VB, Dias A, Hawthorne M, Nirmal Kumar B (2011) Introduction of a new surgical technique: minimally invasive video-assisted thyroid surgery. Clin Otolaryngol 36:51–56
16. Miccoli P, Pinchera A, Materazzi G, Biagini A, Berti P, Faviana P, Molinaro E, Viola D, Elisei R (2009) Surgical treatment of low- and intermediate-risk papillary thyroid cancer with minimally invasive video-assisted thyroidectomy. J Clin Endocrinol Metabol 94:1618–1622
17. Bellantone R, Lombardi CP, Raffaelli M, Boscherini M, Alesina PF, Princi P (2002) Central neck lymph node removal during minimally invasive video-assisted thyroidectomy for thyroid carcinoma: a feasible and safe procedure. J Laparoendosc Adv Surg Tech A 12:181–185
18. Brunt LM, Jones DB, Wu JS, Quasebarth MA, Meininger T, Soper NJ (1997) Experimental development of an endoscopic approach to neck exploration and parathyroidectomy. Surgery 122:893–901
19. Naitoh T, Gagner M, Garcia-Ruiz A, Heniford BT (1998) Endoscopic endocrine surgery in the neck. An initial report of endoscopic subtotal parathyroidectomy. Surg Endosc 12:202–205
20. Huscher CS, Chiodini S, Napolitano C, Recher A (1997) Endoscopic right thyroid lobectomy. Surg Endosc 11:877
21. Yeung HC, Ng WT, Kong CK (1997) Endoscopic thyroid and parathyroid surgery. Surg Endosc 11:135
22. Ballantone R, Rombardi CP, Raffaelli M (1999) Minimally invasive, totally gasless video-assisted thyroid lobectomy. Am J Surg 177:342–343
23. Shimizu K, Akira S, Tanaka S (1998) Video-assisted neck surgery: endoscopic resection of benign thyroid tumor aiming at scarless surgery on the neck. J Surg Oncol 69:178–180
24. Shimizu K, Akira S, Jasmi AY et al (1999) Video-assisted neck surgery: endoscopic resection of thyroid tumors with a very minimal neck wound. J Am Coll Surg 188:697–703
25. Shimizu K, Tanaka S (2003) Asian perspective on endoscopic thyroidectomy: a review of 193 cases. Asian J Surg 26:92–100
26. Ikeda Y, Takami H, Sasaki Y, Kan S, Niimi M (2000) Endoscopic neck surgery by axillary approach. J Am Coll Surg 191:336–340
27. Ohgami M, Ishii S, Arisawa Y, Ohmori T, Noga K, Furukawa T, Kitajima M (1999) Scarless endoscopic thyroidectomy: breast approach for better cosmesis. Surg Laparosc Endosc Percutan Tech 177:342–343
28. Yamashita H, Watanabe S, Koike E, Ohshima A, Uchino S, Kuroki S, Tanaka M, Noguchi S (2002) Video-assisted thyroid lobectomy through a small wound in the submandibular area. Am J Surg 183:286–289
29. Miccoli P, Bellantone R, Mourad M, Walz M, Raffaelli M, Berti P (2002) Minimally invasive video-assisted thyroidectomy: multiinstitutional experience. World J Surg 26:972–975
30. Miccoli P, Berti P, Raffaelli M, Materazzi G, Baldacci S, Rossi G (2001) Comparison between minimally invasive video-assisted thyroidectomy and conventional thyroidectomy: a prospective randomized study. Surgery 130:1039–1043
31. Gough IR, Wilkinson D (2000) Total thyroidectomy for management of thyroid disease. World J Surg 24:962–965
32. Zhang W, Jiang ZG, Liu S, Li LJ, Jiang DZ, Zheng XM, Shen HL, Shan CX, Qiu M (2011) Current status of endoscopic thyroid surgery in China. Surg Laparosc Endosc Percutan Tech 21:67–71

33. Ishii S, Ohgami M, Arisawa Y, Ohmori T, Noga K, Kitajima M (1998) Endoscopic thyroidectomy with anterior chest wall approach. Surg Endosc 12:611
34. Ikeda Y, Takami H, Sasaki Y, Takayama J, Niimi M, Kan S (2003) Clinical benefits in endoscopic thyroidectomy by the axillary approach. J Am Coll Surg 196:189–195
35. Kang SW, Jeong JJ, Yun JS, Sung TY, Lee SC, Lee YS, Nam KH, Chang HS, Chung WY, Park CS (2009) Gasless endoscopic thyroidectomy using trans-axillary approach; surgical outcome of 581 patients. Endocr J 56:361–9
36. Chung YS, Choe JH, Kang KH, Kim SW, Chung KW, Park KS, Han W, Noh DY, Oh SK, Youn YK (2007) Endoscopic thyroidectomy for thyroid malignancies: comparison with conventional open thyroidectomy. World J Surg 31:2302–2306
37. Camarillo DB, Krummel TM, Salisbury JK (2004) Robotic technology in surgery: past, present, and future. Am J Surg 188:2S–15S
38. Lobe TE, Wright SK, Irish MS (2005) Novel uses of surgical robotics in head and neck surgery. J Laparoendosc Adv Surg Tech A 15:647–652
39. Bodner J, Fish J, Lottersberger AC, Wetscher G, Schmid T (2005) Robotic resection of an ectopic goiter in the mediastinum. Surg Laparosc Endosc Percutan Tech 15:249–251
40. Lee J, Kang SW, Jung JJ, Choi UJ, Yun JH, Nam KH, Soh EY, Chung WY (2011) Multicenter study of robotic thyroidectomy: short-term postoperative outcomes and surgeon ergonomic considerations. Ann Surg Oncol 18:2538–2547
41. Lee S, Ryu HR, Park JH, Kim KH, Kang SW, Jeong JJ, Nam KH, Chung WY, Park CS (2011) Excellence in robotic thyroid surgery: a comparative study of robot-assisted versus conventional endoscopic thyroidectomy in papillary thyroid microcarcinoma patients. Ann Surg 253:1060–1066
42. Lee KE, Rao J, Youn YK (2009) Endoscopic thyroidectomy with the da Vinci robot system using the bilateral axillary breast approach (BABA) technique: our initial experience. Surg Laparosc Endosc Percutan Tech 19:e71–e75
43. Miyano G, Lobe TE, Wright SK (2008) Bilateral transaxillary endoscopic total thyroidectomy. J Pediatr Surg 43:299–303
44. Landry CS, Grubbs EG, Morris GS, Turner NS, Holsinger FC, Lee JE, Perrier ND (2011) Robot assisted transaxillary surgery (RATS) for the removal of thyroid and parathyroid glands. Surgery 149:549–555
45. Kang SW, Lee SC, Lee SH, Lee KY, Jeong JJ, Lee YS, Nam KH, Chang HS, Chung WY, Park CS (2009) Robotic thyroid surgery using a gasless, transaxillary approach and the da Vinci S system: the operative outcomes of 338 consecutive patients. Surgery 146:1048–1055
46. Kang SW, Jeong JJ, Yun JS, Sung TY, Lee SC, Lee YS, Nam KH, Chang HS, Chung WY, Park CS (2009) Robot-assisted endoscopic surgery for thyroid cancer: experience with the first 100 patients. Surg Endosc 23:2399–2406
47. Kang SW, Jeong JJ, Nam KH, Chang HS, Chung WY, Park CS (2009) Robot-assisted endoscopic thyroidectomy for thyroid malignancies using a gasless transaxillary approach. J Am Coll Surg 209:e1–e7
48. Koh YW, Park JH, Kim JW, Lee SW, Choi EC (2010) Endoscopic hemithyroidectomy with prophylactic ipsilateral central neck dissection via an unilateral axillo-breast approach without gas insufflation for unilateral micropapillary thyroid carcinoma: preliminary report. Surg Endosc 24:188–197
49. Ikeda Y, Takami H, Sasaki Y, Takayama J, Niimi M, Kan S (2002) Comparative study of thyroidectomies: endoscopic surgery versus conventional open surgery. Surg Endosc 16:1741–1745
50. Kang SW, Lee SH, Ryu HR, Lee KY, Jeong JJ, Nam KH, Chung WY, Park CS (2010) Initial experience with robot-assisted modified radical neck dissection for the management of thyroid carcinoma with lateral neck node metastasis. Surgery 148:1214–1221
51. Lee KE, Koo do H, Kim SJ, Lee J, Park KS, Oh SK, Youn YK (2010) Outcomes of 109 patients with papillary thyroid carcinoma who underwent robotic total thyroidectomy with central node dissection via the bilateral axillo-breast approach. Surgery 148:1207–1213

52. Singer MC, Seybt MW, Terris DJ (2011) Robotic facelift thyroidectomy: I. Preclinical simulation and morphometric assessment. Laryngoscope 121:1631–1635
53. Lee J, Yun JH, Nam KH, Choi UJ, Chung WY, Soh EY (2011) Perioperative clinical outcomes after robotic thyroidectomy. Surg Endosc 25:906–912
54. Lee J, Lee JH, Nah KY, Soh EY, Chung WY (2011) Comparison of endoscopic and robotic thyroidectomy. Ann Surg Oncol 18:1439–1446
55. Yi O, Yoon JH, Lee YM, Sung TY, Chung KW, Kim TY, Kim WB, Shong YK, Ryu JS, Hong SJ (2013) Technical and oncologic safety of robotic thyroid surgery. Ann Surg Oncol 20:1927–1933
56. Lee J, Nah KY, Kim RM, Ahn YH, Soh EY, Chung WY (2010) Differences in postoperative outcomes, function, and cosmesis: open versus robotic thyroidectomy. Surg Endosc 24:3186–3194
57. Perrier ND (2012) Why I, have abandoned robot-assisted transaxillary thyroid surgery. Surgery 152:1025–1026

The manufacturer's authorised representative in the EU is Springer Nature Customer Service Centre GmbH, Europaplatz 3, 69115 Heidelberg, Germany. If you have any concerns regarding our products, please contact ProductSafety@springernature.com

Printed and bound by CPI Group (UK) Ltd, Croydon, CR0 4YY

25/03/2026

02078169-0013